8 to Your
IDEAL
WEIGHT

RELEASE YOUR WEIGHT & RESTORE YOUR POWER IN 8 WEEKS

MK MUELLER

For permission requests, please contact the publisher at:

Mango Publishing Group
2850 Douglas Road, 3rd Floor
Coral Gables, FL 33134 USA
info@mango.bz

For special orders, quantity sales, course adoptions and corporate sales, please email the publisher at **sales@mango.bz**. For trade and wholesale sales, please contact Ingram Publisher Services at **customer.service@ingramcontent.com** or +1.800.509.4887.

Library of Congress Cataloging
Names: Mueller, MK
Title: 8 to Your IdealWeight / by MK Mueller
Library of Congress Control Number: 2016918121

ISBN 9781633534810 (paperback), ISBN 9781633534827 (eBook)

BISAC Category Code: HEA010000 HEALTH & FITNESS / Healthy Living

Front Cover Image: Illustrations designed by Freepik
Author Photograph: Sebrie Images Photography

8 to Your IdealWeight: Release Your Weight & Restore Your Power in 8 Weeks
ISBN: 978-1-63353-481-0
Printed in the United States of America

"Blending her decades of experience as life coach and author with the best of self-help wisdom, MK Mueller has created a simple how-to guide for becoming our Ideal selves. Her powerful 8-step process offers a path for readers to not only release weight, but to follow their passion and discover their personal greatness."

- Dr. Francois Sauer, MD.,
author of Relearn, Evolve and Adapt and advisor for the SHINE program at the Harvard School of Public Health

"My work in wellness has taught me that you must heal the heart before you can fully heal the body. MK Mueller's approach to regaining your wellbeing is about so much more than losing weight. It is about listening to and honoring your body, mind and heart. If you're ready to create lasting change in both your weight and wellbeing, then this brilliant book with simple yet powerful steps will get you there."

- Dr. Michelle Robin,
Wellness chiropractor and host of the Small Changes, Big Shifts podcast, and founder of Your Wellness Connection

"On 8 to Your IdealWeight I am NEVER hungry, yet I've released 35 pounds and I am at a weight I haven't seen in years. I'm happier than I can remember and have SO MUCH MORE CONFIDENCE! Each day is better than the one before – there's no stopping me now!"

- Mary R.

"Obsessive exercise, calorie counting, low fat diets, protein shakes, even working part-time at a women's fitness center... I tried it all! Weight control has been a significant part of my adult life, but I didn't realize that it was all the heaviness in my head that I had to release first! The emotional baggage I had been carrying for years was weighing me down. Today as I write this, my tears of appreciation for this incredible program are rolling down my cheeks and onto a physical body of which I can be proud. Thank you to 8 to Your IdealWeight for giving me my life back!"

- LeAnn F.

"We come into this program thinking that releasing the weight will solve our problems, then discover that solving our problems releases the weight."

- Lorri C.

TABLE OF CONTENTS

Foreword...............................10

Chapter 1

Getting Started.........................11

My Journey.............................12

The Three Prongs of 8 to Your IdealWeight....20

Prong I: Real Food.....................25

Prong II: Real Self-Love..............29

Prong III: Real Connection............42

Chapter 2

The 8 to Your IdealWeight Program.........48

Making the Food Program Work For You......49

The S.A.A.B. Food Guidelines..............53

Your S.A.A.B. Grocery List................58

Chapter 3

The Power Pyramid.....................64

Stepping Back Into Our Power..........65

Chapter 4

The 8 High-Ways Process. 77

The 8 High-Ways Overview. 78

High-Way 1: Get the Picture. 83

High-Way 2: Risk 92

High-Way 3: Full Responsibility. 107

High-Way 4: Feel All Your Feelings. 131

High-Way 5: Honest Communication. 149

High-Way 6: Forgiveness of the Past. 163

High-Way 7: Gratitude for the Present 180

High-Way 8: Hope for the Future 197

How to Become a Certified IdealWeight Coach. . .202

Chapter 5

Additional Resources. 203

IdealMeals and Snacks 204

How to Stay on Program While You
Travel/Vacation. 212

How to Stay on the S.A.A.B. Program When
Eating Out. 214

How to Break Through a Plateau. 215

Acknowledgments

Author Bio

FOREWORD BY PAM GROUT

On my blog, I write a series, "Why I'm the luckiest person on the planet." Last I checked I was up to Episode 24. One of the reasons I feel so blessed is because I meet the most amazing people. My possibility posse attracts really awesome people. People who inspire me, people who are doing life-changing things.

MK Mueller is one of those people. When she stumbled into our Sunday group (well, she didn't actually stumble), I knew right away that this was someone I wanted to know. She spoke truth. She spoke miracles. She spoke love.

And as I've gotten to know her, my respect for her has only grown. She's doing big things. She's making a difference. She's shepherding in the more beautiful world we all know is possible.

I'm honored to write this foreword for her new book. I can say wholeheartedly that her 8-step IdealWeight process based on her 8 to Great book is well, great. And I know that anyone who gets within range of MK is going to be catapulted into a whole new way of living.

Thanks, MK, for your life-changing wisdom and, most importantly, for never wavering, never failing to walk the talk.

Pam Grout,
#1 New York Times bestselling author of E-Squared,
E-Cubed, Thank and Grow Rich and 15 other books

Chapter 1

Getting Started

MY JOURNEY

In August 1986 I was lost. The counselor on the phone had just told me I was in a domestic violence marriage and that my life was in danger. Then she gave me the address of a shelter where my daughter and I would be safe.

My denial was thick, but I had too many secrets to share them with anyone else, so I trusted that she knew what she was talking about and packed up a few things for us. After my husband left for work the next day, we left.

That month-long program changed my life forever. Where my degree with honors from a prestigious university had given me knowledge, my counselors at the shelter gave me wisdom.

Four weeks later, as I re-entered my world, I didn't want to forget what I'd learned about honoring and standing up for myself, so I decided to start a support group. I put notes in 10 neighbors' mailboxes, inviting them to my living room on a Saturday morning for the very first "Taking Care of Me" class. Five people showed up that day, and although none of them were in a domestic violence situation, the empowerment message resonated with all of them.

Soon I was hosting classes in church basements and small businesses, regularly hearing the same request: "Please put this in a book." My reply that I wasn't "a writer" got weaker as time went on, and eventually my first book, **"Taking Care of Me: The Habits of Happiness,"** was published.

The journey from those early days of watching women and men reclaim their happiness and personal power to today as a Life Coach and International Keynote Speaker has been a glorious one. For the past three decades, I've been coaching people of all ages - from business leaders and educators to CEO's and Moms groups - to happier and more successful lives through my 8-step process, *"8 to Great."* Today I'm so proud that over 2500 PowerCoaches are living and sharing that process around the world.

So in January 2014, life was good. I lived every day in gratitude, but also in fear. I woke up every day afraid of what I might eat, and went to bed every night guilty about what I'd eaten. I wasn't consuming food, food was consuming me.

Meanwhile, what my audiences didn't see on stage was that my energy was low and getting lower. Getting through a day of speaking wore me out. Playing tennis after a day of writing was just not an option, and I watched my life become more and more sedentary. My weight continued to increase, but I couldn't bring myself to go back to counting calories or points. I attributed it all to getting older, and resigned myself to believing it was inevitable.

It was at that point that my chiropractor and friend, Michelle Robin, D.C., suggested I consider a dietary change - **release sugar's hold on me.**

"But I don't get sick!" I challenged, dreading the thought of having to give up my fast food breakfast and daily dose of diet soda. What I didn't tell her was that I was successful at only one thing with diets - failing. I had tried every weight loss gimmick available for 30 years. Like 90% of women, I'd gone on more than 16 crazy calorie-counting and point-counting diets in my 30's, 40's and 50's. None of them had been sustainable.

"You'll feel and look years younger, MK. Just give it a try for 2 weeks."

I trusted her, so I watched the documentaries **"Fed Up"** and **"That Sugar Film."** I was stunned when I found out how the big food industries had stacked the cards against us by putting addictive levels of sugar in almost every processed food.

Instead of getting depressed, I got mad. I had been the "Sugar Queen" who had to have my favorite candy every day and had been tricked into a life of fat and fatigue. I trusted the mountain of new research findings - that if I just gave my body a few days to "detox," and started checking food labels for added sugars instead of calories or fats, I would be on my way to a lifetime of freedom.

I purchased the hottest new diet book on lowering my added sugar intake and gave it a try. (I remember feeling really dizzy for the first 24 hours. My body's detoxing really took it out of me, so I was glad I'd chosen a weekend to start it.)

But there was a problem. Over those next two weeks I could barely keep up with all the "rules." The diet didn't just limit my added sugars, it required 10 daily supplements, 30 minutes of exercise each day, daily detox baths, a media fast, no dairy, no caffeine, keeping records of sleep, food intake, etc. I told my friends it felt like a part-time job just trying to remember it and get all my homework done.

By the 14th day, I had released 7 of the 20 pounds I wanted to lose and I had no sugar cravings, (no small miracle!) but the rest of the program was just too much. I couldn't sustain it.

Within a month I had gone back to my old ways and gained back the weight.

I felt like a failure again, and I was angry.

I knew that removing added sugars was good for me. Why couldn't someone offer a program that was easy, that worked in everyday life for normal people, and that would be a way to eat for life rather than for a few high-deprivation months?

That day I went back to my notes, got out my scissors and started cutting. I would test a food plan that **did** allow dairy and caffeine so I could have butter and cheese and drink my morning cup of coffee with cream. What did I have to lose but my belly fat, fatigue and mood swings?

Within 8 weeks on this incredibly simple program, I released 20 pounds while enjoying the most delicious food I'd ever tasted. Eating real food was not only easier than I believed, but all of a sudden it tasted like a banquet.

The Email that Birthed this Book

What happened next was much more than a coincidence. I got an email from one of my readers. Jim had heard me speak years before and wrote to thank me. In his email he shared how, when he was on the brink of absolute despair, the 8 steps of my *8 to Great* book had helped him find the courage to get healthy, release 150 pounds, and turn his life around. He got me thinking.

I knew that releasing sugar addiction was the only sustainable way to release weight without cravings, and that most people believed it was impossibly difficult. I also knew that my 8-step process would supply the motivation to stay the course as new habits were developed. I decided to test a blend of my simple 4-step sugar awareness program with my equally simple *8 to Great* process.

Today I not only have hundreds of success stories, but scores of Certified Coaches of this process around the world who are helping women and men achieve the same amazing and sustainable results.

And now it is with great gratitude and joy that I am sharing this powerful process with you.

Here we grow!

MK

The First Step in Your Journey to Your IdealWeight

You are reading this now because you are considering a powerful change. With this program, change will come your way immediately, not just in how you relate to food, but how you relate to feelings, to family, and to your reflection in the mirror.

This process won't just change how you eat. It will change how you feel about yourself.

So if change is what you're looking for, you've made a great choice.

This program is based not only on the newest information on the epidemic of addiction to added sugars, but also on my 30 years of learning, living and coaching a proven process for aligning our hearts and minds.

I call that process "The 8 High-Ways" because it will get you on the road to success faster and get you where you want to go. Picture an iceberg.

Now imagine that the peaks above the surface are your "problems." One might be money, or relationships, or a job you don't like, but the big one is **weight**. "If only I could lose this weight," you keep thinking, "then I could be happy."

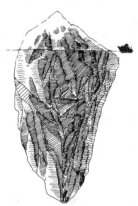

So you go on diet after diet, chipping away at that one peak. Maybe even making some progress, but it **never helps.** Why? Because all the ice underneath the surface keeps attracting and freezing more ice on top.

Here's the good news:

> 1. *This program will take a huge sledge hammer to what's below the surface, helping you release regrets, self-doubt, worry, and all other thought forms that lead to unhappiness, addictive eating patterns, and an 'ice-olated' life.*

> 2. *Once the underlying issues are released, not only will the extra weight fall away for good, but so many other issues in your life will start to clear up, from indecision ... to debt ... to clutter, and more.*

"We come into this 8 to Your IdealWeight program thinking that releasing the weight will solve our problems, then discover that solving our problems releases the weight."

- Lorri C.

What this healing requires is your focus and coachability for 8 full weeks.

The Challenge - Finding Your Balance

I believe I know something about you. If you're like most people reading this, you take better care of others than you do yourself. It's time to balance the scales. So as your Coach, here is my first challenge:

Put yourself first. For 8 weeks make taking care of You the prime focus. What's the worst thing that could happen if you rebalanced your priorities for that short amount of time? Whatever it is, it pales in comparison to your potential for creating an amazing life six months or a year from now.

You are worth this time. If you weren't, you wouldn't have come off the Heavenly production line. You deserve happiness by being here, and it's time to claim it.

Meanwhile, in return, I promise that I will keep this process simple, because *if a concept isn't simple, it is impossible to remember and therefore impossible to use.* Therefore, you won't be asked to count points, calories, carbs or steps. I am regularly thanked for creating "the simplest food program ever!" and believe that simplicity is the key to its success.

Through **8 to Your IdealWeight**, you'll be joining a community of women and men who, after completing the program, are some of the happiest and healthiest people I know..

On this program you will learn:

- *Why diets don't work.*
- *That the 1980s "low fat" movement resulted in the industrial food industry tripling and quadrupling the amount of added sugars in food.*
- *That sugar is 8 times more addictive than cocaine and added sugars are used in many foods we think of as healthy options.*
- *That the dramatic increase in obesity and diabetes is due to the sugars added by the food industry, not from eating fats or lack of exercise.*
- *The influence the food industry wielded in the absence of reporting requirements for added sugars on food labels.*

"Food is being intentionally manipulated by the top 12 food industries. Their foods are designed to create cravings and addiction. Sugar addiction is the root cause of why people are overweight and sick today."

- Dr. Mark Hyman,
author of "The Blood Sugar Solution"

Imagine feeling free of cravings after just **one week** of lowering your added sugars to healthy levels (18 g. or less per day). These are some typical results our participants have shared after following the program.

- *Cravings for sweets disappeared*
- *Inflammation and joint pain were dramatically reduced*
- *Energy to spare for the first time in years*
- *Fewer headaches, backaches, colds and flu viruses*

- *Discovered new healthier ways to be comforted without food*
- *Noticed clearer thinking and sharper memory function*
- *Real food tasted good again. Really good.*
- *Belly fat and scale numbers decreased weekly with no hunger*

The Three Prongs of 8 to Your IdealWeight

Because this program will help you live your IdealLife, I'll be referring to you from now on as "**Ideal.**"

Our **8 to Your IdealWeight** tagline is: **Get Real. Get Healthy. Get Empowered.** As I've mentioned, it's about healing so much more than our food issues. We will **Get Real** - not just with food, but also with ourselves and each other. There are 3 prongs to this process, and all are equally important.

The 3 Prongs of the 8 to Your IdealWeight Program:

I. A Program for Weight Release Focused on Real Food

II. A Personal Empowerment Process for Real Self-Love

III. A Partner for Real Connection

I. Real Food

You'll learn why diets don't and can't work, how fat doesn't make us fat, sugar does, and how you can, like I did, release the hold that added sugars have had on your health once and forever *without cravings, hunger, or feeling deprived.*

Meanwhile, you'll discover how delicious Real food (the unprocessed kind) can taste! I succeeded with this program because it didn't require cooking skills, raw salads or smoothies. Instead, it offered a banquet of delicious, inexpensive and easy-to-prepare options.

I promise that once you stop hijacking your taste buds with highly addictive sugary foods, Real food will taste so good and sweet that you won't crave anything else. That may be hard to believe, but it's true.

II. Real Self-Love

After being released from the brain fog, fatigue, joint pain and despair of sugar addiction, we'll start on an 8 High-Ways journey - learning to love ourselves and follow our dreams that have been locked away.

When I first revealed the 8 High-Ways Process in my book *8 to Great*: **The Powerful Process for Positive Change**, it won numerous awards and was hailed by best-selling authors like Mike Dooley as "powerful from cover to cover, revealing the greatest secrets that have ever been shared."

This personal empowerment process is designed to help you...

- *reconnect with the dreams you thought you had lost*
- *honor your feelings instead of numbing them with food*
- *make decisions that are the right ones for you every time*
- *learn to communicate in more authentic and assertive ways*
- *discover a powerful positive attitude formula to savor every day to the fullest*

More than just the *ingredients* of a happy life, you will also be given the *recipe.*

III. Real Connection

One of the strongest prongs of our program is our very active and engaged online community. You have the option to join us. If you do, you'll select your very own IdealWeight Coach, be supported by and get to know your support group of 10 other individuals on the program, and select or be assigned one Ideal from your small group to partner with. To find a coach or join a small group, go to www.8toyouridealweight.com.

If you don't choose to journey with a coach or small group, it is essential that you find your own partner to Get Real with for this journey.

Either way, you'll be sharing four things with your partner each week for 8 weeks:

- *Texting or emailing a checkin on eating breakfast, staying on the food program, etc.*
- *Texting or emailing 3 new daily Gratitudes, with no repeats*
- *Texting or emailing a weekly photo of your feet on the scale for your weight check-in*
- *Sharing a weekly phone call to discuss your Reflection Questions from each chapter*

Each section of this book will offer Reflection Questions for journaling to share with your partner. Answering these questions will be as important to your success as releasing added-sugar foods. Through the questions, you'll have the opportunity to Get Real with each other about food, about how you're really feeling, what you're really thinking, and who you're really dreaming of becoming.

"After releasing 40 pounds, I have seen firsthand how reaching out and sharing with my partner and my group has affected my release and my attitude. I couldn't have done it without their support."

- Linette M.

This 3-pronged program began as an engaged and enthusiastic small group of 10. Today there are thousands of participants being coached by *8 to Your IdealWeight Certified Coaches* around the world. Individuals come looking not only to release their weight, but to restore their power, as Cathy did.

Cathy's Story

Cathy decided to commit to the process after a conversation over lunch. It was a beautiful fall day, and I had just given a seminar at her workplace. As we sat down to eat, she commented on my food choices, noticing I wasn't eating the bread on the sandwich. "If I follow your program, will I eat like that?" she asked with a bit of a grimace.

"Yes," I replied. "And you will not only fall in love with food instead of being afraid of it, you will almost never feel hungry."

She rolled her eyes and laughed. She couldn't yet imagine what she'd be writing me just six months later...

"I feel so blessed to have been on this journey with 8 to Your IdealWeight. I have learned so much about myself through this life-changing process. This week I was able to buy birthday treats for my daughter without feeling the need to partake! I love the feeling of having power over food instead of food having power over me. I like to tell people my weight release of 40+ pounds to reach my IdealWeight

is a very happy side effect of learning to love myself. Many thanks to MK, my partner and our small group. Today I'm truly living my IdealLife!"

As Cathy demonstrates, our journey together will not only end your cravings for sugary sweets, it will also build a clear path back to self-love. As we release the shame, guilt, regrets, blame, worry, fear and limits that we have worn as a wall of protection around our bodies, our freedom and power will return. With them will come a strong inner confidence - and the assurance that nothing can ever take our power away again.

PRONG I: Real Food

Releasing Our
Sugar Addiction

Let's start by asking the question:

Am I Addicted to Sugar?

Answer "Yes" or "No" to each item below.

1. Do I feel compelled to drink diet or regular-sugared soft drinks throughout the week, often going out of my way to get them?

☐ Yes ☒ No

2. Do I find myself thinking about sweets and desserts, or even anxious if they're not served?

☐ Yes ☒ No

3. Do I regularly wake up groggy or hit a mid-afternoon energy slump?

☐ Yes ☒ No

4. Am I unable to resist bread or salsa chips on the table at a restaurant?

☒ Yes ☐ No

5. Do I find myself feeling guilty after eating certain foods, and/or sometimes eating even more out of guilt?

☒ Yes ☐ No

6. Do pictures or even talking about sweets trigger my cravings?

☑ Yes ☐ No

7. Do I find myself reaching for every candy dish I pass?

☐ Yes ☑ No

8. Am I unable to have sweets or desserts in the house without dipping into them?

☑ Yes ☐ No

9. Do I have trouble stopping after one bite of sweets or chips?

☑ Yes ☐ No

10. Do I find myself eating certain foods even when I'm not hungry because of cravings?

☑ Yes ☐ No

If you checked "Yes" more than once, don't be discouraged. Freedom from sugar addiction awaits you through this powerful process.

Note: When participants start our 8-week program, their average score is 9 out of 10 Yeses. After they complete 8 weeks or more, their average score is 1 out of 10.

The Top 10 Reasons Sugar Isn't Sweet

1. It is addictive - 8 times more than cocaine - making us want more and more and more.

2. It causes inflammation and joint pain.

3. It turns to belly fat, the most dangerous fat storage for our health.

4. It is the leading cause of obesity in America, which is one of the fastest growing causes of death in the U.S.

5. It is the leading cause of diabetes, the prevalence of which has doubled in the past two decades. Diabetes left untreated can cause kidney disease, blindness, heart disease, neuropathy, stroke or even death.

6. It creates "brain fog," which prevents clarity and mental awareness.

7. It rots our teeth.

8. It causes fatigue from blood sugar spikes and drops that make us tired just an hour after a full meal.

9. It overrides Leptin, a hormone that acts as an "I'm full" indicator switch, leading to overeating due to never feeling full.

10. It promotes wrinkling and aging skin.

These are just the top 10. There are dozens more, including a 40 percent increase in despair and depression impacting millions like you and I every day.

As Lynn wrote in a fun Facebook post, sugar is anything but sweet.

> *"I realized I was ready to shed the full length 'cover-up' I was wearing to the beach. Thanks to 8 to Your IdealWeight, my belly fat is now out of my 'Protection Collection.' That outfit was so last year!"*
>
> *- Lynn M.*

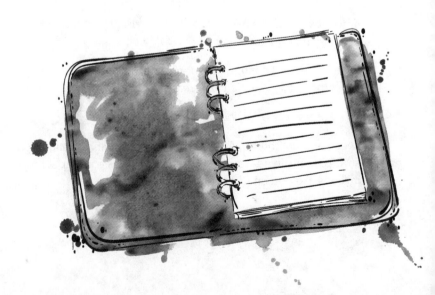

PRONG II: Real Self-Love

The Lies We Believe

In the past, we have believed the lies that we were "less than" or "not enough." These lies poisoned us, and led to our running to food for comfort.

The good news is that lies are just lies. They have no power over us, and when brought to the light of awareness, they cannot survive.

It's time for you to take back your power by seeing yourself for who you truly are, a bright light who is worthy of the greatest respect and love, able to do and be anything as you follow your heart.

Take a moment to review the following limiting beliefs to see where you may have given your power away in the past. Put a check next to the beliefs that feel familiar to you:

- ☑ I can't lose weight.
- ☐ I'm not worth it.
- ☐ I don't deserve it.
- ☑ My metabolism is slow.
- ☐ Healthy food doesn't taste good.
- ☑ Healthy food doesn't fill me up or satisfy me.
- ☐ I always gain the weight back.
- ☐ I can't do food programs because I don't like to/ have time to cook.

☐ Thin people are all stuck up anyway.

☐ I hate exercise.

☐ If I release weight, I'll just sabotage myself.

☐ If I lose weight I'll be vulnerable.

☐ I can't afford to buy new clothes.

☒ Sweets are an important part of our family traditions.

☐ If I lost weight my spouse would want sex all the time.

☐ Programs like this take too much time.

☐ I don't like eating breakfast.

☒ It is too much effort to cook separate meals for my family and me.

☐ Eating healthy is too expensive.

☒ I won't be able to enjoy going out with my friends on the program.

☒ My work schedule is too crazy right now.

Now write out a response to counter each of the above statements you selected. Write down the truth you know about each limiting lie. For example:

LIE: Programs like this take too much time.

A Possible Counter: *If I added up how much time I spend looking online for the next diet, complaining about my weight, shopping for clothes that look decent on me at this weight, going to the doctor, getting my pain meds filled, taking naps because I'm exhausted, etc., it would be obvious that it takes more time to stay at this weight than being healthy ever would.*

The truth doesn't cost you anything, but a lie could cost you everything.

The Power of Commitment - Your Personal Agreement:

We Don't "Find" the Time, We Make It

Mary Beth Helgens and I have known each other since high school. I had followed her career as a health and wellness coach with great admiration. She is someone I look up to for her loving heart, her strong faith, and her incredible courage.

The day she contacted me about going through the program, I was amazed and delighted. I knew how busy and full her life was already, and the fact that she wanted to make time to participate meant a lot. Today, she is one of the program's brightest coaching stars. She made time to be her best self.

"Once I followed these 8 simple steps and stopped craving sweets, I have enjoyed more successes on and off the scale. I couldn't wait to tell my daughter! Since then she also became an Ideal, achieved her IdealWeight, and became an IdealWeight Coach! Transformed by this process, we are empowering others to do the same."

- Mary Beth Helgens,
Certified Health and Wellness Coach and IdealWeight Coach

We have had Moms of four young children who had full time jobs successfully complete this program. If they could do it, so can you.

When your Why is big enough, you will find your How.

Your Personal Agreement

It's time to be really clear on what it is you want and why. Take a few minutes to complete this **Personal Agreement**.

On a separate sheet of paper or in your journal, write out the answers to the blanks below. The answers will help you get started and stay motivated.

1) I resolve to commit to this 8-week **8 to Your IdealWeight** Course so that...

2) My extra weight has been challenging in many ways, including...

3) These challenges have resulted in more problems and issues such as...

4) I am ready and willing to be coached because I have found that the old ways have not worked. This has resulted in feeling...

5) Without help, a year from now I will still...

6) I am ready to reach and maintain my IdealWeight with this program, which will result in my feeling...

7) This will benefit me in so many areas of my life, including...

8) To summarize my Why for choosing this new lifestyle in just a few words, it would be...

9) To do this I am willing to...

10) I deserve and welcome abundant happiness and health because...

I am making this 8-week commitment to myself to Get Real, Get Healthy and Get Empowered in order to live my best life, to release my sugar addiction and guilt about food forever, and to learn to truly love my body and myself.

This is the first day of the best of my life.

_____   _____
DATE   SIGNATURE LINE

Congratulations! Keep a copy of this commitment form in sight for the next 8 weeks. Read it regularly until it's a part of who you are.

The Power of Release - The Goodbye Letter

Ideals, our spirits have been hungry. We have been hungry for acceptance, for love, for respect, for happiness, for forgiveness, and for a sense of worthiness and honor. We have looked for these things in our jobs, our spouses, our children, our parents, our bank accounts and our mirrors, but we still found ourselves starving...for what they could not give us.

We are lovable and we are loved. That is the truth that can nourish and refresh us whenever we remember it. With this knowing, we can courageously confront the lie of not enough - that thief that has stolen our joy and kept us from living our best and sweetest lives.

We haven't just been duped about sugar over the years, but also about our innate worth. If someone told you that you were a genius, would you believe them? Most of us would say, "No." Yet how many of us believe the opposite when someone labels us that way?

The fact is that you *are* a genius. One of the definitions of genius is "a natural ability." Admit it. You have special gifts that no one else on earth has. Your unique life journey, intuition and connection to your Higher Power have given you insights, wisdom and power that you have never fully acknowledged.

Like Simba in **The Lion King** and Elsa in **Frozen**, we have been running away from acknowledging our wisdom and our courage, yet these very gifts have been with us all along.

It's time to use that courage to come home to ourselves - to acknowledge that we have allowed our body and spirits to be abused by sugar, and that sugar has isolated us and made us feel unlovable. Today the abuse ends as we say goodbye to our extra weight and our old habits.

Sugar Was My Abusive Partner

Chelsea, a wife, Mom, speech therapist and 8 to Your IdealWeight Coach saw abuse as a pattern in her life. One she'd never seen in herself...

As I went through the 8 to Your IdealWeight program, I realized how much sugar reminded me of an abusive partner.

Growing up I had a friend who always seemed to pick the worst guys. They were losers who would treat her awful 90 percent of the time; and the other 10 percent when they were half-way decent, it was just to get what they wanted.

Once the abuse started, mentally and physically, I would beg her to stop seeing them. Unfortunately, all I could do was be there for her when she would need comfort after a rough patch. I would tell her over and over how she didn't deserve this, but she always went back because somehow the addictive actions and words of those men were able to get into her head more than I was. It wasn't easy to watch, but I always hoped one day she would get angry enough to stop the cycle.

I can see now that sugar has been an abusive boyfriend to my mind and body. The headaches, body aches, and extra weight were evidence of a sick love affair with sugar - much like bruises from a violent relationship. It treated me badly, and I kept going back because, for a minuscule amount of time, it felt good. The other 95 percent of the time I allowed it to do horrible things. My mind and body have cried out with signals like pain or illness begging me to protect them.

Nowadays I am befriending myself and loving my body. I am learning I deserve so much better and will be so much better off without sugar addicting my body and tainting my amazing mind. I am kicking out my abusive partner.

I have finally broken the cycle of sugar's abuse. The journey this program has taken me on is one for which I am, and will be, eternally grateful.

- Chelsea Phipps,
8 to Your IdealWeight Coach

Facing Ourselves

Your life is about to change. If you have a smartphone or camera, take a "before" selfie of your full body with your clothes on. (In the mirror may work the best.) It will feel good to look back at your "before" pictures down the road. If you feel uncomfortable keeping it, you can always delete it or throw it away.

A Goodbye Letter to Your Extra Weight

There is nothing as powerful as our own words, and it's time to put yours on paper in the form of a goodbye letter.

If you don't have a journal, get some writing paper and a pen. Find a quiet place to sit with a writing surface where you won't be disturbed. If you can, prepare yourself for this writing time by listening to an inspirational song like, "Brave" by Sara Bareilles, "Fight Song" by Rachel Platten, or the gently powerful "Try" by Colbie Caillat.

First decide what or who you will write to. You may write it to your extra weight, acknowledging the purpose it served, and saying a respectful farewell, or you may write it to a particular food that you turned to for comfort in the past.

It may feel uncomfortable at first. Let it. It's perfectly normal to feel anger, sadness, fear, regret or anything else. Just allow your feelings to flow through you as you write. To feel is to heal.

When you're finished with the letter, you can share it with your partner, coach or small group, and then burn it, or burn it immediately. Either way, letting go will help you start this journey with a clear resolve and a heart that's free.

Here is an example of the power of release from an Ideal who eventually released 50+ pounds and reclaimed her freedom:

Dear Extra Weight,

You have been surrounding me and covering me with your soft, jello-like form. On sad days and lonely nights you were all I had, and at the time it seemed like you were my only solace. As I lived with your comforting ways you grew and grew and GREW. Your growth alarmed me and I chose to handle it by not looking in the mirror, telling myself at my age it didn't matter because I had no one in my life to impress anyway. I tried to shrink you and make you go away, but you hung on for dear life and continued to grow. I saw that I had made a huge mistake inviting you in.

You kept me from going out. I was embarrassed to see old friends, knowing they would wonder why I let you join me. I was embarrassed to meet new friends knowing they would not be able to see the true me as you surrounded me so completely that my true identity was hidden. You made me cry...a lot.

Then by a (blessed) chance I met a stranger who told me of a plan that just might send you out the door. That's why I'm giving you a swift kick! Out of my life Extra Weight! I'm releasing you! This is a one-way ticket, no returns! In the next 8 weeks I am going to see your sorry behind disappear for good! I will see you melt away like Frosty the Snowman did on that sunny day. Good riddance and O Happy Day!

- Hanni H.

Now it's time to let your heart speak its truth.

The Butterfly Meditation

Once you have completed and burned your letter, honor the sacred moment of transformation with a deep breath, and if it feels good, spend a few minutes in a cleansing meditation such as this one:

Close your eyes and see yourself stepping into a cocoon that closes around you. Take 8 slow, deep breaths. With each breath, say "I love and accept myself unconditionally." Slowly feel yourself transforming inside the cocoon and experiencing the miracle of metamorphosis into a beautiful butterfly.

Then imagine yourself breaking out of your cocoon, spreading your wings ... and soaring!

Mirroring Your Power - The Mirror Mantra

"My husband just posted this under our photo in our church directory, 'Dale loves Debbie.' I know our renewed romance after all these years is because I finally love me."

- Debbie G.

Next it's time to start your daily **Mirror Mantra**.

In the past, our relationship with mirrors has not always been affirming, and often we avoided them because of the pain they awakened in us. It's time for that to change.

From now on, each morning when you first get up, look yourself in the mirror and take a deep breath. Then, while looking into your eyes, say the words below aloud. When you reach the third phrase, fill it in with **a word that feels good to you that day,** such as "enough," "amazing," "powerful," "worthy," "courageous," "committed," "strong," "transforming," "resilient," "awesome," "my hero," "phenomenal," or "beautiful."

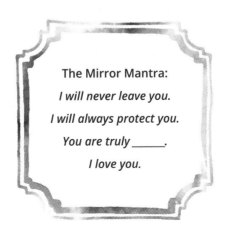

The Mirror Mantra:
I will never leave you.
I will always protect you.
You are truly _____.
I love you.

As you speak this daily mantra, feel the shift of beliefs within you as the days go by. Feel the power of your words as they change your thoughts, your feelings, and your actions.

What you think

⤷ *Determines what you feel*

⤷ *Which determines what you do*

⤷ *Which determines who you are*

Speaking Your Power: Freedom Phrases

As we experience with the Mirror Mantra, our words are powerful. Here are some re-phrases that will refresh our spirits and renew our hope. As you replace the old phrasing with the new, you will reboot how you think and how you feel.

Replace **"I lost weight."**
(You don't want to find it again!)
with **"I am releasing my extra weight."**

Replace naming sugary food items such as,
"I was tempted by the birthday cake."
(When we picture it, we often want it.)
with the word **"sweets."**

Replace "I can't seem to...."
(Your brain believes you!)
with "I haven't yet...."

Replace "I need to..."
(You are all that you need already.)
with "I am going to..."

"Replace "Fat..."
(We're releasing this painful word from our vocabulary.)
with "extra weight."

Replace "I'm on a diet"
(Diets are temporary.)
with "I love my Get Real Program for life..."

Replace "I'll try..."
(The mind hears the word as struggle.)
with "I will..." or "I'll do my best."

Replace "He/She makes me so..."
(No one can make us happy or sad.)
with "I feel a little ___ when she/he/you..."

Replace "I should"
(Don't should on yourself or other people.)
with "I could..." or "I'm going to..."

Replace "This is hard."
(It's as hard as we believe it is.)
with "This is new."
Soon you'll be saying "This is easy."

 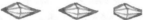

Remember this:

If you wouldn't say it to a friend,
don't say it to yourself.

 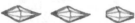

PRONG III: Real Connection

Willpower vs. Willing Power -
Trusting Your Coach

"These days, not only are the scales measuring my success,
but so is the mirror - I can't stop smiling!"

- Melva N.

You have stated that you are ready and willing to be coached. It will make all the difference in your results.

Think back for a minute. Who have been your greatest coaches?

My "Willing" Decision

When my counselors at the shelter told me not to so much as mention my husband's name for four weeks, it was hard. But I reminded myself that if I knew better than they did, I wouldn't have landed myself there.

I noticed the other women in the program ignored the rule, and spoke of their exes every chance they had. As it turned out, I was the only woman out of the seven of us that did not return to a violent relationship. The fact that I was willing to be coached made all the difference.

We always have a choice - with any coaching resource - to trust or not to trust the advice we're given.

When you trust the process in this book, it means that for 8 weeks you'll be all in. It means you'll see me as your Personal Coach and be coachable.

How a Coach Benefits Us

A Coach invites us to do things we would otherwise not do. She challenges us to do things we believe at first we cannot do. With our Coach we step into a new level of courage, first to trust their lead, then to trust our own inner wisdom.

A Coach calls us to commit, to make a promise to ourselves and keep it. Her main concern is not to make us comfortable, but to move us to a new level on the playing field of life, which is often uncomfortable. She knows that real progress takes commitment and perseverance, and that once achieved, it will bring us to a feel-good place that lasts a lifetime.

I have been coaching people of all ages for the past 25 years, and take my responsibility as your coach very seriously. From the days in my 30s as a weight-loss program lecturer, to having trained over 2,500 people as trainers for my *8 to Great* and 8 to Your IdealWeight process, I am excited about getting to coach you now.

The Benefits of a Small Group

If you decide to join the online **8 to Your IdealWeight Community**, you'll be part of a small group of 8-10 under the direction of a **Certified 8 to Your IdealWeight Coach** and select or be assigned a partner within that group. Your weigh-in will be with the Coach instead of your partner.

The advantages of small group membership are numerous. It brings with it a feeling of normalcy. As you hear the stories of others, you'll know you are not alone. You'll share daily encouragements and weekly celebrations. Our Coaches are personally living this program and are as committed as you are to your well-being and success.

In addition to the weekly check-ins with your partner, you'll also receive:

- *A day planner/journal*
- *Daily check-ins with your group on Facebook (see below)*
- *Two live Conference Calls each week*
- *Optional 1-on-1 Coaching with your Personal Coach*
- *An optional Alum Facebook page and weekly newsletters for one year following the 8 weeks*

More information is available at www.8toyouridealweight.com, or by calling 828-242-9033.

Bottom line: whether I am your only Coach, or you reach out to a Certified Coach and small online group for additional support, your success will depend on your willingness to trust.

The Daily Partner/Small Group Check-in

Each day for these eight weeks, email or text your partner with a Y (Yes) or an N (No) for five accountability goals. To help remember them, they're in alphabetical order:

- *F for* **First meal** *if you ate breakfast with some protein. N if you did not. There are many on-program breakfasts in the Resource Section of this book.*

- *F for* **Fitness** *if you moved more than you did before starting this program. This could be as simple as taking the stairs instead of the elevator or walking around the block after dinner.*

- *F for* **Food** *program if you followed the Real Food S.A.A.B. guidelines.*

- *F for* **Freedom** *if you released your excess stuff, items such as clothes, household items or old magazines. **

- *G for sharing 3 new* **Gratitudes** *each day with your partner via email, text, FB messaging, phone or in person. (More in High-Way 7).*

* In all my years of coaching, I've never known someone who wanted to release extra weight that didn't also need to release excess material things as well.

Remember to share your Y's and N's with your partner through email or text every day for these 8 weeks. (In the online class, you'll share them with your entire small group and coach each day.)

First Meal (Eating Breakfast)
Fitness (Moving Our Bodies)
Food Program (Releasing Sugar Addiction)
Freedom (Release of Excess Stuff)
Gratitude (Sharing 3 New Gratitudes Each Day)

 Heartwork in Preparation

1. Watch the documentaries, **"That Sugar Film"** and **"Fed Up"** (the version with narrator Katie Couric). Both are 90 minutes and both can be found on iTunes or Amazon.

2. Clear your cupboards. If your family will prefer to keep off-program foods around, put them on a separate shelf in the refrigerator and in a separate cupboard if possible.

"I always cook for my family on the 8 to Your IdealWeight plan. (I haven't told them and they haven't even noticed a difference - 4 months now!) I regularly get comments from my husband like, 'restaurant quality meal,' 'best meal so far,' and 'this is my favorite.' He now has many favorites and I'm so happy about that."

- Ann S.

 Partner/Reflection Questions

For your initial partner sharing, reflect and/or journal answers to these questions. Then discuss your responses with your partner and/or Coach.

1. Start your first call by discovering 3 things you have in common other than that you're in this program.

2. Where and when do you feel (have you felt) most powerful?

3. When and to whom do you sometimes give your power away?

4. Share your answers to these questions:

> How will your testimonial read once you successfully reach your IdealWeight?

> How will your IdealLife feel at your IdealWeight?

5. If you're willing, share your Goodbye letters with each other.

"I can only be loved as much as I allow myself to be known. As long as I hide, if someone says they love me, my ego whispers, 'They wouldn't say that if they really knew you.' And then we don't let love in."

- John Maxwell,
author of *"How Successful People Think"*

Chapter 2

The 8 to Your Ideal Weight Program

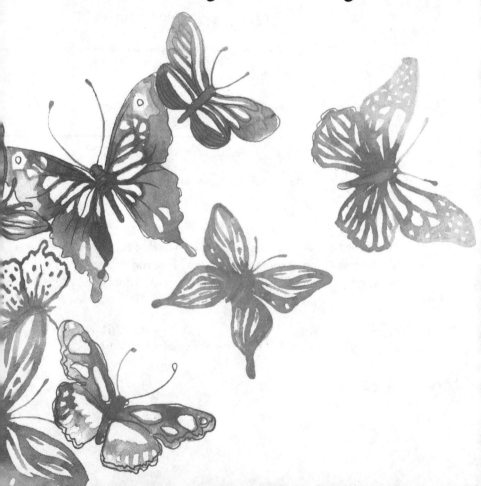

MAKING THE FOOD PROGRAM WORK FOR YOU

"I've released my first 20 pounds and the best part is I no longer think, 'I can't wait until I can have this again,' because I don't even want that stuff any more. I've found a new healthy lifestyle based on delicious real foods and I know I will stick with it for a lifetime!"

- Katy L.

I'm about to ask you to replace some of your favorite foods with foods that you'll fall in love with within a week or two. Can you do it? Of course you can. The only question is how quickly.

Every person is different. Some Ideals ease into this program, spending a week eating the last of their off-program foods and cleaning out their cupboards before they get started. Others make all the changes in one day. You get to decide.

If you're one who would like to make changes gradually, start with these 12 Replace-to-Release options on your own timetable:

12 Replace-to-Release Options

1. Replace fruit juices with real fruit.
(Avoid dried or sugar-added fruits such as Craisins.)

2. Substitute sweet potatoes for white potatoes.
(A good-sized sweet potato takes just 6 minutes to cook in the microwave. Add all the butter and cinnamon you want, and within a week it will taste like dessert.)

3. Replace ice cream with 1/4 c. of whipped cream, real fruit and nuts (cinnamon optional). (My favorite is Reddi Wip original dairy whipped topping.)

4. Replace flavored coffees or artificial sweeteners in your coffee with 1 tsp. of table sugar and real cream. (One tsp. of sugar is about 4 grams.)

5. Replace artificial sweetener on your oatmeal with two chopped dates. (Steel Cut oatmeal is preferred.)

6. Replace chips with Mary's Gone Crackers or nuts.

7. Replace diet or regular sodas with tea (+ 1 tsp. table sugar you add yourself), Perrier, or LaCroix flavored waters. (They will taste sweeter every day that you're on program.)

8. Replace bread with lettuce wraps (a la Jimmy John's unwich) or simply release bread completely. (You will be so full and so satisfied after every meal, you'll wonder why you ever traded your waistline for sandwiches.)

9. Replace eating pizza with eating pizza toppings. (You'll enjoy 3-5 pieces of pizza toppings, not feel stuffed or tired after the meal, and release weight the next day!)

10. Replace alcohol with Perrier or San Pellegrino when you're eating out. (Sometimes I'll even drink it from a wine glass!)

11. **Replace chocolate bars with low sugar Kind bars.** (Be sure to check the label and only select the ones with 6 g. or less of sugar in each bar, and limit yourself to one per day.)

12. **Replace desserts with a piece of sugar free gum after your meals.** (Most have just trace amounts of artificial sweeteners.)

S.A.A.B. Full Program General Guidelines

1) **KISS: Keep it Simple Sweetheart!** This program limits added sugars, **not** calories, fats, or fiber. Release any need to check calories ever again. That will only slow down your progress. An easy, although oversimplified way to remember this is, "Fat makes us thin. Sugar makes us fat." We promise this program will get you off sugar addiction and cravings for good!

2) **A Get Real Food Program for Life.** This is not a "First this, but later that" food program. **It offers one simple program for life.** Real food will soon taste so good, you won't ever want anything else.

3) **No Measuring, just Mindfulness.**

Alcoholics Anonymous (AA) has an acronym - **H.A.L.T.**

For this program, we add an "s" - **H.A.L.T.S.**

Instead of Measuring, we use Mindfulness and ask ourselves: Am I Hungry? Angry? Lonely? Tired? Sad?

It is healthy to eat between meals. I encourage it. Simply be aware - if one handful of on-program foods satisfies you, then you were Hungry. When you find yourself wanting more than one handful, you're either:

Angry - You could journal or have a talk with someone.

Lonely - You could call someone or join a meetup on *www.meetup.com.*

Tired - You could take a nap, shut off media earlier, or go to bed earlier.

or **Sad** - You could journal, rest, or contact a friend.

One handful of nuts, a little cottage cheese and fruit, a cheese stick, or a few gluten-free crackers will satisfy you if it's hunger you're feeling.

4) Get Real. Get Healthy. Get Empowered. This "Get Real" program recommends eating whole, unprocessed foods whenever possible. Choose real foods, such as sliced roast beef instead of bologna or a hotdog, real cream for your coffee instead of creamer, and Swiss cheese rather than highly processed American cheese.

NOTE: If you suffer from any medical conditions, such as high blood pressure, before starting, be sure to check your personal food program with a nutritionist, your primary care physician, or a medical professional. Blood pressure has been known to decrease significantly on this program, and needs to be monitored for those who have had issues or are under a doctor's care for this condition.

THE S.A.A.B. FOOD GUIDELINES

S.A.A.B. stands for the 4 food groups we release or reduce:

Sugar - Artificial Sweeteners - Alcohol - Bread

SUGAR (You may enjoy 5-6 grams added sugar* per meal maximum)

Examples of high sugar foods we release:

- *Sweet drinks: all fruit juices, sweet teas, sugared lemonade or waters, diet and regular sodas, tonic waters, etc.*
- *Sugar added foods: candies, desserts, many salad dressings or yogurts, etc.*
- *Low-fat anything (because sugar amounts are tripled or quadrupled when fat is removed)*

*You can check for added sugar by the ingredients list. A package of frozen blueberries may indicate 12 g. of sugar per cup, but those are natural sugars within the fruit because the only ingredient is "blueberries." If, however, the package ingredients include any of the sugar names, then count all sugar grams as added sugars.

Limiting sugars to 5-6 grams per meal (1 tsp. table sugar or honey) or a total of 18 g. per day, means recognizing its many names: fructose, sugar, corn syrup, honey, corn sweetener, cane sugar, dextrose, fruit juice, brown sugar, etc. Be sure to read labels on all your foods, including salad dressings and balsamic vinegars, yogurts, tomato sauces, canned fruits, protein or breakfast bars, and bacon.

The Good News: You'll be amazed at how delicious and sweet regular foods taste once you get off these incredibly high sugar foods. Two weeks after starting, a girlfriend invited me over for lunch. She made a wonderful spinach salad with feta cheese, almond slices and strawberries. When I tasted the fruit I blurted out,

"You added sugar to these strawberries?"

"Of course not. Why would I do that?"

"But these are so sweet. Are you sure?"

"I rinsed them before adding them, MK. I'm sure!"

Then we both laughed, realizing that I was finally cleared of high sugar foods and artificial sweeteners and could enjoy real food for the first time in decades!

I've heard this experience described by hundreds of Ideals. Within a week or two most do not miss high sugar food at all. Can you imagine the freedom you will feel when you get there?

ARTIFICIAL SWEETENERS

Aspartame (Equal or NutraSweet), Sucralose (Splenda), Saccharin (Sweet'n Low), Neotame. These mock sugars are 40-400 times sweeter than sugar. Hijacking your taste buds with *any* artificial sweeteners is delaying your ability to taste the natural sweetness of foods. Once you fully release artificial additives then fruits, vegetables and sweet potatoes will taste like desserts and added sugar foods will soon taste "sickeningly" sweet.

Note: We also eliminate plant-derived sugar substitutes on S.A.A.B. such as xylitol, stevia and agave, as they overstimulate our tastebuds and therefore raise our cravings for highly sweetened foods.

The Good News: If you're like many of us, getting off diet soda and the mindset that "it doesn't hurt me because it's low calorie" is one of the hardest shifts to make. Be patient with yourself as you would with a potty-training child. You may choose to cut down slowly or cease sodas all at once.

One tip: When I'm on the road and driving through a fast food pick up lane to get scrambled eggs and bacon (which I can get all day every day almost anywhere in the US), I always request a free cup of water. I love the fact that it comes iced with a straw. It "feels" a lot like my soda used to and is easy to drink while I'm driving.

Eventually the day came when I had *no* desire for a diet soda, but be patient, this one may take 2-4 weeks.

ALCOHOL

- *Beer*
- *Wine*
- *Hard Lemonade*
- *Hard Apple Cider*
- *Liquor*

The Good News: This is a hard and fast rule for the first 8 weeks because consumption of alcohol lowers your resistance to those old temptations. But once you have your first 8 weeks under your belt, you may choose to enjoy some wine or a beer as part of your daily 18 g. of added sugar option.

BREADS

- *Breads*
- *Pasta*
- *Rice*
- *White Potatoes*
- *Corn*

When we eat carbohydrates, our digestive system breaks them down into sugar that causes a blood sugar spike, which creates an insulin surge, which causes a blood sugar crash, which causes all the other problems. Even whole wheat bread is mostly devoid of any real nutrients, and most of the brands have high fructose corn syrup added. It's a shock at first to release "sandwich" from your vocabulary, but after a week or two, it can feel like a game - one where you are always the winner!

The Good News: The good news here is that bread will be easier to release than you think. Once you get used to taking the bread off sandwiches and enjoying the meats, cheeses and veggies all rolled up, or asking for the bowl of steak and veggies at Chipotle's with sour cream and guacamole, you'll feel full without feeling stuffed. You'll leave the meal ready to dance through the day rather than having to go home and take a nap!

Heart Disease - America's #1 Cause of Death

It is worth noting that the (AHA) American Heart Association recently updated their added sugar intake recommendations, reducing them dramatically. As of 2015, the recommended added sugar intake for adult women is 6 teaspoons (24 grams) per day. Adult men's recommended added sugar intake is no more than 9 teaspoons (36 grams).

"Naturally occurring sugars in fruits, vegetables, and dairy don't need to be avoided; they make up part of a healthy diet."

- Rachel K. Johnson,
Professor of nutrition at the University of Vermont in Burlington and one of the experts who came up with the AHA guidelines.

The New Way to Read Labels

In the spring of 2016, the government (F.D.A.) decided that sugar awareness was important enough to change our food labels. It was a clear sign that the country was finally responding to the research on the dangerous impact of added-sugar foods.

The New Food Label: What's Different?

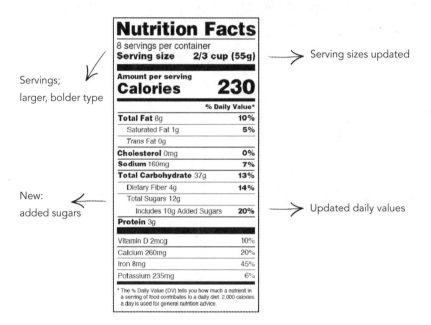

Servings; larger, bolder type

New: added sugars

Serving sizes updated

Updated daily values

On this program we never check labels for calories or fat content, only for sugars (before 2017) or added sugars (with the new labels 2018 on). It is a dramatic new behavior for most of us, and one that will free you from your worry, guilt and extra weight!

YOUR S.A.A.B. GROCERY LIST

Grocery List Options for the S.A.A.B. Food Program

Don't just read the labels, read your body. Everyone's body is different.

Have fun enjoying the following foods while avoiding or limiting Sugar, Artificial Sweeteners, Alcohol, and Breads:

ALL VEGETABLES

___Artichokes

___Beets

___Broccoli

___Brussel Sprouts

___Carrots

___Cauliflower

___Celery

___Cucumbers

___Eggplant*

___Fresh Garlic

___Green Beans

___Kale

___Mushrooms (Portobello)

___Onions

___Peppers

___Romaine Lettuce

___Spinach

___Sweet Potatoes

___Squash

___Tomatoes*

Note: * Technically a fruit.

ALL FRUITS

___Apples
___Apricots
___Avocados
___Bananas
___Blueberries
(frozen or fresh)
___Coconuts
___Cuties Oranges
___Dates*
___Grapes
___Grapefruit
___Mangos

___Oranges
___Peaches
___Pears
___Pineapples
___Plums
___Prunes*
___Raisins*
___Raspberries
(frozen or fresh)
___Strawberries
___Watermelon

(Note: fruit juices are NOT on S.A.A.B.)

*Raisins, Prunes and Dates are dried fruits with no added sugar and may be eaten with portion awareness. Dried pineapples, bananas, Craisins, etc. almost always have added sugar and are not on program.

ALL UNPROCESSED MEATS

___Chicken
___Beef
___Lamb
___Pork
___Turkey

Avoid highly processed meats such as hot dogs, lunch meats, etc.

ALL FISH

___Bass

___Cod

___Flounder

___Grouper

___Haddock

___Halibut

___Mahi Mahi

___Marlin

___Orange Roughy

___Red Snapper

___Redfish

___Salmon

___Scallops

___Sole

___Tilapia

___Trout

___Tuna

___Yellowtail

ALL EGGS

(Rather than just eating the white, enjoy the entire egg!)

OILS

___Butter

___Coconut Oil

___Extra-Virgin Olive Oil

___Avocado

___Coconut Butter

___Olives

___Almond Butter

NUTS AND SEEDS

___Almonds

___Cashews

___Chia seeds

___Flax Seeds

___Macadamia nuts

___Pistachios

___Pumpkin Seeds

___Quinoa

___Sesame Seeds

___Sunflower Seeds

____Pecans   ____Walnuts
____Pine Nuts

(See peanuts under "Limited Legumes")

DAIRY

____All naturally cultured Cheeses (not highly processed)

(Processed cheeses include American Cheese, cheese in spray cans, cheese spreads, etc. If it says "cheese food," "cheese product," "cheese spread," or "made with real cheese," it is not cheese. For example, Velveeta is not made of cheese.)

____Milk (Whole and 2% are preferred over skim)
____Plain Yogurt
____Sour Cream
____Cottage Cheese
____Real Whipped Cream

MISCELLANEOUS

Be especially aware of portions and how your body reacts to the following:

A SWEET OR CHOCOLATE OPTION: Kind Bars with 6 g. or less of sugar are allowed. (At this printing there were five that fit that category.)

LIMITED LEGUMES: This category means we eat them with heightened portion awareness. Watch how they impact your energy and your weekly release and make your best decisions. Legumes include such foods as black beans, peas, peanuts, snap peas, chickpeas, lentils, hummus, alfalfa, tofu, etc.

CAFFEINATED DRINKS: Flavored or Plain Coffees and Teas are acceptable. Check to make sure that no sugars or sweeteners are added.

SPICES: All Spices are acceptable. Be aware that iodized table salt often contains trace amounts of sugar.

BRIDGE FOODS AND BEYOND: Just as it may take weeks to release diet soda from your life, in my early sugar awareness days I chose to eat 1/3 c. oatmeal made with steel cut oats for breakfast with real fruit, nuts, cinnamon, chia seeds and flax or hemp seeds for extra protein.

Enjoying oatmeal with no added sugars for breakfast has been an option for me and many successful Ideals since then. Just keep in mind that weight releases and energy levels may improve with a higher protein breakfast.

Likewise, early in my program, I was missing a crunchy food, and discerned that Mary's Gone Crackers was my healthiest option. While they do contain some brown rice, they are full of nuts and seeds. Again, it's all about finding what works for your body.

NOTE: If your grocer doesn't have what you're looking for, ask for it!

Our 4 IdealWeight Inner Releases

We no longer have a need for these four: Guilt, Hiding, Impatience and Judgment.

To help you release these four habits that do not serve you, take a minute to read the following aloud to yourself and affirm:

There are no bad foods, no bad scale numbers, no bad decisions. I release the need to ever feel **guilt** about anything within my value system again. I can say "No" without guilt, and "Yes" without guilt. I am always doing the best I can and what I need to do at that moment, for reasons known or unknown. It is all perfect.

I no longer need to **hide**, because the world is a safe place. I have friends and coaches I am open and honest with, as they are with me. Openness allows my connection to them and to myself. I am safe.

Everything happens in Divine timing, so I release my **impatience** and unrealistic expectations. I am comfortable with my journey, complete with its ups and downs, detours and seeming dead-ends. Everyone is my lover or my teacher. I grow from both. And for every door that closes, another one, to an even better place, always opens.

I release the need to **judge** myself and others for any reason. When I sense that others are judging me, it is a reminder that perhaps they are my mirror, and I have some self-judgment to release. Meanwhile, I release my judgment of those who are at a different place along their journey than I am in mine.

Finally, I take invitations to change for just that, invitations. And like any other invitation, I accept them when and how I feel comfortable, on my terms, and on my timetable. All is well.

Every day I am releasing. It is a natural process that cannot be stopped. Every day I am receiving. It, too, is a natural process. I am enjoying them both!

Chapter 3
The Power Pyramid

STEPPING BACK INTO OUR POWER

"We do not need magic to transform our world. We carry all of the power we need inside ourselves already."

- J.K. Rowling,
author of the Harry Potter series

Now that you're aware of sugar's harmful impacts, let's talk about how to step back into your personal power - the power you've had all along, but may have forgotten how to use.

Is power a good thing? Of course. Your eyes are using power to read these words right now. Power is like electricity, it is inherently a very good thing, but there are bad things we can do with it. And the worst thing we can do with our power is to give it away.

The Power Pyramid

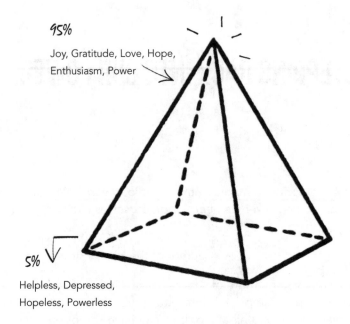

95%

Joy, Gratitude, Love, Hope,
Enthusiasm, Power

5%

Helpless, Depressed,
Hopeless, Powerless

Imagine that your level of power at any given time could be charted on a Power Pyramid.

Then imagine that when you choose thoughts that feel good, like joy, gratitude, and love 95% of the time, you are hovering near the top at a 95 out of 100, and feel powerful. We'll call that "95ing" because you're using 95% of your power.

On the other hand, when we give our power away to thoughts that don't feel good, like regret, shame, worry, judgment or fear, we can feel helpless and hopeless. We call this hovering at the bottom of the Power Pyramid "5ing" because you're only using 5% of your power.

Another way of saying it is that when 95% of your thoughts feel good, you are "95ing." When only 5% of your thoughts feel good, you are "5ing."

At the bottom of the Power Pyramid, what goes around comes around, and you will attract other "5ers" because misery loves company.

The great news is that joy loves company also, and when 95% of your thoughts feel good, you will attract other "95ers."

Feeling Powerless Over Food

For decades, I knew the pain of feeling powerless over food. All that time I was I beating myself up mentally because I thought I "should" be able to change my eating habits. No matter what successes I had professionally, I used my weight as an excuse to feel out of control.

And then one day, everything changed. I remember it like it was yesterday. It was the day I decided to feel my anger (or "angergy" as we'll call it in this program) and take my power back over food. I vowed that I would find the key to turning around my thoughts and commit to changing my eating habits once and for all.

Nothing has been the same since. Every single aspect of my life has been transformed for the better. And let me be clear - the shift did not come from my being a certain dress size. It came from owning my power and choosing thoughts that felt good.

Why is it so important to choose thoughts that feel good? Because when we do, we feel good.

When You Feel Good

Why is it so important to feel good? Take a minute to ask yourself this question and come up with half a dozen of your own answers....

"When I feel good I..." (For example, "I have more energy.")

Answers like "I smile more," "I laugh more," or "I'm more patient" often show up on this list. You may have written, "I'm kinder, more creative, and more productive."

If you took the time to write down all the hundreds of possible answers, you'd see that **everything you've ever wanted in life would end up on this list.** And where did all these gifts come from? Not from being at our goal weight or from winning the lottery.

They came from feeling good, which came from choosing thoughts that feel good. To sum up this amazingly simple truth:

1. When you choose thoughts that feel good, you feel good.

2. When you feel good, good things happen.

"Neither losing weight, finding a soulmate, writing a book, nor becoming a billionaire will ensure happiness. Nothing ensures happiness. No dream come true will do. Because happiness that's not present at the start of a journey will not be present at its end."

- Mike Dooley,
www.tut.com

Happiness is not the destination in life, happiness is the way. And it starts with one thought at a time. What are you thinking right now? Notice how that feels.

Your Daily Gratitude Homework:

How we start our day is one of our most important decisions, so I'm giving you **homework for every day for the rest of your life.** (Note: Only do this on the days you want to feel good. Don't do it the other days.)

Starting tomorrow, somewhere in your morning routine, share 3 new things you're grateful for with someone through email, text, Facebook messaging, phone or in person.

Then do that each day while following one more rule: **No repeats.** That's right. If you're grateful for sunshine tomorrow, you're done with sunshine for life. :)

This simple daily ritual is tremendously transforming, shifting our focus from what went wrong each day to the myriad of blessings we received. As an Ideal wrote to me early in her program,

> *"I can't believe it's just been a month since I started this program. Simple things like thinking of my gratitudes throughout the day and I'm a completely changed person. I came here for weight help and now my marriage has improved and I have more energy. Wow!"*

> \- Connie B.

All that for an investment of less than one minute a day.

When Problems Seem Too Big

If your life is maddening and messy right now, it may take some extra effort to find the gratitudes hidden in each day. Here's a true story that may help.

In 2010, Haiti was going through a painfully slow rebuild after 200,000 people lost their lives in an earthquake. My dear brother Jim, a dentist, flew there to volunteer for two weeks. I later discovered that he pulled over 50 teeth a day from the mouths of Haitians, and that their rotted teeth were the result of chewing on sugarcane. I also heard stories of very little clean air or water, and a lack of infrastructure from government offices to schools.

So you can imagine my surprise when my brother's first words to me on the phone when he returned were, "MK, you won't believe how grateful they are."

What did the Haitians possibly have to be grateful for?

- *They were alive. (We've got that one too, right?)*
- *The whole world was coming to help them.*

We can all agree that if the Haitians could find things to be grateful for, those of us with clean air, clean water, and 5,000 choices at our local supermarket can do the same.

Your gratitudes could be as simple as:

- *"I'm grateful I can choose to be grateful."*
- *"I'm so grateful for the sound of my loved one's voice on the phone."*
- *"I'm grateful for my ten toes inside the shoes on my feet."*

We'll talk more about the Gratitude Ritual in High-Way 7.

"I'm so grateful for the daily gratitudes: I shared three with my husband and daughter yesterday for the first time, and before I could even ask if they wanted to share their gratitudes, they both jumped right in!"

- Ann S.

How Long Does It Take to Move Back up the Power Pyramid?

No matter what is happening in your life right now, it is your choice whether or not you surrender your power to it. Feel your feelings, while focusing on thoughts that feel good. Instead of watching the news tonight, go for a walk.

Instead of asking someone "What's new?" ask him or her to share the best part of their day. Instead of posting and liking angry Facebook posts, post beautiful or inspiring ones. Choose what you feed your mind.

You'll be amazed at what a difference small changes can make. We are never sitting still on the Power Pyramid. We are always moving either up or down. So how long does it take to shift your position on the Power Pyramid? As long as it takes you to think your next thought.

Our Most Important Job

Your most important job today, and every day, is the same as mine -- choosing thoughts that feel good! No matter what happens around us, what is happening within us is what matters most.

"We must remind each other that everyone who is a queen simply knew she could be one. That's all that separates the queens from the slave girls; a shift in consciousness from denial to acceptance of personal power... We can't look to the world to restore our worth; we're here to restore our worth to the world. The world outside us can reflect our

glory, but it cannot create it. It cannot crown us. Only God can crown us, and He already has."

- From "A Woman's Worth" by Marianne Williamson

Redefining Selfish

Dear MK,

My word for this year is "receive." At first glance it might seem rather selfish, but I decided that I wanted to open myself to the gifts that the universe had to offer.

In January I signed up for my first 8 weeks of 8 to Your IdealWeight with Coach Sue Fitzgerald. How rich are the gifts I have received! I am a trimmer, healthier self with a wonderful support system of strong, vulnerable and compassionate women. The journey has been challenging as I've been guided to explore old hurts and release grudges. I am a work in progress.

Thank you for creating this program. I am blessed and will continue to be open to receive all the lovely things the universe has in store for me.

Love,
Marilyn B.

I wanted to share a bit of Marilyn's beautiful letter because I'd like to propose a re-definition of a misaligned word: **selfish**.

Consider this reframe: hiding our gifts under a bushel basket of fear is selfish. Not asking for what we want is selfish. Self-caring behaviors are never selfish - quite the opposite.

Choosing self-caring behaviors is the most loving thing we can do for ourselves and others.

For 44 Ways to "Take Care of Me" go to www.8toyouridealweight.com/recipes4life

How We Lost a Genius

The week I was writing this chapter, I saw the movie *"The Man Who Knew Infinity."* It is the true story of a mathematical genius who changed that field while still in his 20s.

The movie theme is a painfully common one. He did not want to bother his mentor, G.H. Hardy, with his need for the special vegetarian food that aligned with his religious beliefs; so while living at the University of Cambridge in London amidst lavish wealth, he often went to bed hungry. As a result of poor nutrition, a severe vitamin deficiency, and a myriad of other dreadful living conditions, Srinivasa Ramanujan's immune system was weakened, and he died at an early age of tuberculosis, with most of his genius untapped.

How loving were his acts of self-deprivation? Who lost the most when he didn't ask for what he wanted? We all did.

Growing up, I was taught that it is unloving to act without considering the needs of others. I agree. But I was never taught how unloving it is to act without considering our own needs. I taught that to myself.

Following our inner promptings, taking care of our needs and following our God-given dreams is not selfish; it is self-loving. Self-love nourishes our hearts and bodies. The more we have, the more we have to give.

"But I have been programmed to put the needs of others first," I often hear from Ideals. Dear Ones, how can we possibly know what others need when we are hardly in touch with our own needs? Meanwhile, if we are waiting for everyone else to be happy before we allow ourselves to be happy, we will go to our graves miserable.

"Love your neighbor as yourself."

The beautiful teaching of Jesus above could also be written as an equation. "Love your neighbor = Love yourself." Are you in balance? If you're taking better care of others than you are yourself, you will soon have little to give. The results can be exhaustion, physical and mental depletion, and eventual resentment toward those who cannot hear what you are not saying.

Starting today, give yourself permission to love yourself as you love your daughter or your niece. Feed her breakfast, give her warm baths, let her take naps, read her love stories, buy her something beautiful, and make sure she gets hugged. The world will be a better place for it.

Redefining Pride:
Half Jerk - Half Jewel

Another word I've seen misunderstood is **pride**. Growing up many of us were taught that pride was the most grievous of sins. Instead, I believe that Love-based pride is the complement to Love-based Humility.

In *8 to Great* I wrote that we are all half-jerk and half-jewel. When we understand that Love-based Humility is the belief, "I'm no better than you," then we can see that Love-based pride is the understanding that, "I'm no worse."

Imagine a world where our children could freely take Love-based pride in themselves. With a companion emotion of Love-based Humility, there would be no desire to put another human being down as being "less." It's a beautiful picture, isn't it?

After I got out of the shelter, I realized that living my life to please others and believing I wasn't good enough had put my life in a danger. It was imperative that I learned to love myself.

So the day came when *I decided to live the kind of life I wanted my daughter to live when she was my age.* I now make decisions from that perspective, and it has served me well for three decades.

What Will Be Your Legacy?

When I ask parents in my audiences, "If you had only one gift to give your children, what would you want it to be?" the answer is always one word, "Happiness."

They're watching.

Modeling happiness for our children is one of the greatest legacies we can leave.

Right now, you have the ability to choose happiness. Once you give yourself permission, I promise this powerful process will take you there. You will see life through new eyes, as Megan described in her thank you note....

"Thanks so much, MK! I am the happiest now that I have ever been. This past year since going through the program has been truly transformative. I feel grateful, blessed, and excited for the future. Truly, your guidance and the wisdom in the 8 to Your IdealWeight program have changed my life!"

- Megan B.

Chapter 4

The 8 High-Ways Process

THE 8 HIGH-WAYS OVERVIEW

The High-Ways are the result of my research into what the happiest, healthiest and most successful people in the world have in common - how they think and act differently from the other 90% of the world...

The Recipe for Happiness

My first book on this subject was *"Taking Care of Me: The Habits of Happiness."* For years, I traveled the world giving presentations on it. But one day a middle-aged gentleman in recovery from his addiction to alcohol walked up to my book table and said, "There's a process in you."

I asked what he meant.

"You're giving us all the ingredients, but we need the recipe for happiness. You need to write that book."

Three months later the tragedy of 9/11 stopped everything. As a result, my regional and national convention keynotes were canceled, and I was able to use that time to write a step-by-step manual for happiness, mental health and success, *8 to Great*: The Powerful Process for Positive Change.

In all the years since, I've never been tempted to add a High-Way to the original 8 or delete one. I am so grateful to be able to share this comprehensive process for "getting where you want to go" with you now.

High-Way 1: Get the Picture

Visualizing the outcome you desire until it feels good is the first step to any dream or goal. Once you're clear on your destination, keep thinking about it until you feel excited about what it will be like. Then, from that good-feeling place, the next step will reveal itself as surely as the next yellow brick showed up on Dorothy's road to Oz. Visualize yourself enjoying wearing shorts in the summertime, easily hiking up that big hill, or traveling the world at your IdealWeight.

High-Way 2: Risk

Once your dream starts to take shape, your next step is taking a risk to follow it. Cowards have the same amount of fear as heroes, but while cowards use their fear as an excuse to stay stuck, heroes feel the fear and do it anyway. Whether it's the risk of telling the truth or pursuing a dream, the bigger the risk, the bigger the reward. Risk is never running from (our fears), it's always running to (our dreams).

High-Way 3: Full Responsibility

As we travel down the Risk High-Way, obstacles and detours will inevitably appear. We can blame and complain about our bad luck, but not without being pulled off course. Full Responsibility is when we acknowledge that we are the biggest problem we have, and therefore we are the solution. Until we see that we are in charge of our lives, we can feel trapped in a prison of resentment, bitterness and confusion. When we acknowledge the power of our thoughts, beliefs and actions, we discover our key to freedom!

High-Way 4: Feel All Your Feelings

As challenges arise, allowing ourselves to feel all our feelings returns us to the freedom of childhood, when emotions came and went without guilt or denial. When we realize that there are no "bad" feelings, we stop suppressing them and getting stuck. We can feel mad and sad and still have a positive attitude. Once we are freed up emotionally, we feel better physically as well. As we overcome the fear and judgment of our own emotions, we can more easily accept the feelings of others.

High-Way 5: Honest Communications

Once we get in touch with our emotions through High-Way 4, we are ready to practice communicating them honestly with others in a self-responsible way. The practice of non-defensive listening and assertively asking for what we want empowers us as well as deepens our connection to those around us.

High-Ways 6, 7, 8: The FGH Formula

The sixth, seventh, and eighth High-Ways make up the world's most powerful positive attitude formula. Because attitude is mental, not emotional, and because all thoughts are either about the past, present, or future, we only need to practice three kinds of thoughts: FGH.

High-Way 6: Forgiveness of the Past

...is knowing we were all doing the best we could at the time with the information we had.

High-Way 7: Gratitude for the Present

...is focusing on acknowledgment and appreciation of the good in every person and situation in the present moment.

High-Way 8: Hope for the Future

...is keeping our eyes on the light of possibilities within us, no matter how small, that helps us persevere through the darkness. It's knowing that our destiny awaits us, if we'll just keep on keeping on.

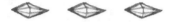

HIGH-WAY 1: GET THE PICTURE

The Power of the Dream

We are heart-wired to follow our dreams. To deny our dreams is to live a life of drudgery, deadlines, and quiet desperation. When we're young, we dream our biggest dreams, but as we age, we often minimize them into small "achievable" goals. That's when life gets hard.

Over the years, I have found that there are deeply personal, yet universal reasons why we want to achieve our IdealWeight:

- *so we can believe in ourselves again*
- *so we can love ourselves again*
- *so we can follow our dreams*

> *"Having a dream is awesome. Having a dream and showing up every day, even when nothing seems to be happening, is priceless. But having a dream and showing up every day, while sauntering, winking and hugging everyone, is when the floodgates begin to tremble."*
>
> - Mike Dooley,
> www.tut.com

When 90-year-olds are asked their top regret, it's always, "I wish I'd had the courage to live my life the way I wanted and not how others wanted me to live it." They regret the dreams they did not follow and the risks they did not take.

You may be thinking your dreams died a few dress sizes ago, but dreams never die. They just get buried underneath fear, guilt and shame. The good news is that your dreams are not dead and buried. They are alive and well. Together, we'll find them again.

"Your time is limited, so don't waste it living someone else's life... Don't let the noise of others' opinions drown out your own inner voice."

- Steve Jobs,
Co-founder of Apple Computers

First let's clearly define what a dream is. I once heard a high school teacher refer to a dream as "an unachievable goal."

What a sad misunderstanding.

It was my dream to write a book (this is my fifth), to have children despite the doctors telling me I couldn't (I have two miracles in my daughter and son), and to put out my own music CD (I now have four CDs full of my original music).

And I'm just getting warmed up. If you're going to trust me on anything, dear Ideals, trust me on this:

All of your dreams are achievable.

"We're never given a dream without the power to make it come true."

- Richard Bach,
author of *"Jonathan Livingston Seagull"*

Dreams are gifts we are given, and they are essential to the **IdealWeight** process. Simply having a goal of "staying on program" will eventually become stale and unsustainable. Staying connected to your dreams – keeping your eye on the prize - will carry you to the freedom and fulfillment you desire.

So how do goals compare to dreams?

Goals are S.M.A.R.T.: Specific, Measurable, Action-oriented, Realistic and Time-based.

Goals are those results we roll out of bed for. They just don't get us excited. Think perspiration. With a Goal we know the Where, When, Who, What, Why and How of what we want.

Dreams are our heart's desires. Your dreams live deep within you. They're what we jump out of bed for. Think inspiration. With Dreams, we ignore Where-When-Who-How and only focus on the What (we want) and Why (because it will feel good).

Because we don't know the "How" with dreams, our imagination must take the lead. We release knowing how it will happen and "Get the Picture" of the end result.

How old were you when you were really good at imagining? Most people say 4 or 5. And then were you told to "Get your head out of the clouds"... "Be realistic"... "Stop daydreaming"? In this program we are returning to daydreaming again, realizing it's the first step to success.

"Ask for what you want, and be prepared to get it."

- Maya Angelou

Michael's Miraculous Medals

U.S. Swimmer Michael Phelps was the first ever athlete to compete in five Olympic Games. When he was interviewed after winning his 8th gold medal (the most medals won by an individual in one Olympic Games), he was asked to share how he was feeling. His reply did not mention his mother, his coach, or his teammates. He knew exactly the message he wanted to send to the world:

"I just want to say how grateful I am for my imagination."

- Michael Phelps

The "facts" as the experts reported them pointed to the physiological impossibility of his feat. They claimed it could not be done. His imagination released the "How" of his dream and took him to the feeling of standing in the famous photograph with 8 medals around his neck. He imagined how it would feel, and as a result, achieved the "impossible."

If you are willing to be happier and bring your sacred dreams to life, you must enter the world of imagination.

Imagine-Nation

Who lives in this nation? All the greats of the world. Everyone from Gandhi, to Martin Luther King, to Walt Disney, to Oprah, to comedian Jim Carrey, to author J.K Rowling. Now I do, too. Won't you join us?

I remember hearing my young son singing non-stop, and I loved every note. Night and day, the most beautiful songs came from his sweet voice. As a young mother, I had a dream of him singing in the *Vienna Boys' Choir* some day and wrote it in my journal, even though we lived in Omaha, Nebraska, at the time.

Within one month of my journal entry, we heard about a prestigious children's choir in the Omaha area. Zach auditioned and was accepted into The Nebraska Choral Arts Society's **Bel Canto** as their youngest member. Later that same year, they traveled to Wales for an international competition, where they finished 3rd, ahead of the *Vienna Boys' Choir.* (You can go to Youtube.com and type in "Z.

Randall Stroope Bel Canto Psalm 23" for a taste of their angelic music.)

If my "impossible" dreams can come true, why can't yours?

"Imagination is more important than knowledge."

- Albert Einstein

Imagine That

High-Way 1: Get the Picture means using our incredibly creative imagination to

Think it 'til we feel it.

Take a moment to think of something you expect to be easy. For example, when planning a trip to a neighboring state, you first save money and then make reservations. The day of your trip you pack up the car, set your GPS, and arrive safe and sound for a fun getaway. That was easy.

Now think of something you **expect** to be hard. Is it finding a partner to walk with? Finding meals on program that your family loves? Releasing your next 10 pounds? How much better would it feel to imagine them as easy? Desire is the accelerator of your dreams. Doubt is the brakes.

"The one who thinks he can and the one who thinks he can't are both right."

- Henry Ford

What we think about we bring about. So the most important, yet often most challenging component of success, is **believing** it will happen. So let's be clear what a belief is...

A belief is a thought you keep thinking until you feel it.

Can you imagine having the energy to run a 5K? Being a role model for fitness to the young people in your life? Feeling comfortable in a swimsuit?

Most people will tell you that they have dreams, but if their dreams exist only in their heads and not in their hearts, it is the same as buying a lamp, setting it on the table, and leaving it unplugged. There will be no light.

When you use your imagination to **believe** in something, you get a sense of how it would look and feel to accomplish that dream. When you start to feel anticipation and get excited, you are connecting with your heart. You've now plugged in the lamp. Voila! The light goes on.

"Everything you pray for, believe that you have it already, and it will be yours."

- Mark 11:24

The CBA Formula

The formula for "Get the Picture" is simple, as simple as ABC, only backwards:

Conceive it.
Believe it.
Achieve it.

Most people stop at Conceiving and never get to Believing their dreams will come true.

Ask yourself, what is the worst thing that could happen from your believing in a dream? You could be disappointed. But then, you have been disappointed many times in life and survived, right?

And what is the best thing that could happen? You would get to experience your dreams coming true; thereby realizing you have a formula for changing your life that you can share with the world.

How much more power could you possibly have?

> *"What you think about is what you talk about, and that is what will come about."*

> — Wenday Cooper,
> Life Coach

 Heartwork for High-Way 1

Create a Dream Board to help you "Get the Picture" of the things you want to attract into your life. There are dozens of website programs that will help you create one online. Or if you're like me, you can get a piece of poster board and a glue stick, and use pictures downloaded from the internet or cut from magazines.

Meanwhile, find a favorite photo of yourself to place in the center. If you have one of when you were at your IdealWeight, use that. If not, use a head shot that you like. Finally, consider writing the words, "I Am Fit and Healthy at My IdealWeight!"

If dreaming big feels like a stretch right now, imagine that someone gave you $100,000 and three months of vacation. What would you do? Where would you go?

Here are some questions to get your imagination warmed up...

Is your dream to:

- *be able to wear your wedding ring again?*
- *have a lap for your kids to sit on?*
- *play catch with your grandkids at the park?*
- *go dancing and feel your partner's hand around your waist?*
- *be back at your wedding weight?*
- *wear a swimsuit on a Caribbean cruise?*

"Thank you! After 11 years, my wedding dress fits again!"

- LeAnn F.

When finished – you'll always be updating it – place it where you'll see it each day, i.e. near the bathroom mirror or in your walk-in closet. Then text a picture of it to your **Ideal** Partner or post it on your **IdealWeight** Facebook page!

"There is no use trying" said Alice. "One can't believe impossible things."

"I dare say you haven't had much practice," said the Queen. "When I was your age, I always did it for half an hour a day. Why, sometimes I've believed as many as six impossible things before breakfast."

- Lewis Carroll,
author of *"Alice Through the Looking Glass"*

 Partner/Reflection Questions

For your sharing this week, consider discussing the following:

1. What great dreamers have I been blessed to meet?

2. I am willing to let myself dream again because...

3. Some of my dreams are...

4. A place I could put my dreamboard where I'd see it every day would be...

"When I first started applying the 8 principles of this book, my life changed dramatically. I not only released weight and started running again, I met the man of my dreams and we've been married for six blissful years. The 8 to Your IdealWeight process works, as so many success stories have proven."

- Amy Krance-Wendt,
8 to Great Master Trainer

HIGH-WAY 2: RISK

Run To, Not From

Krissy was a mom of two young boys, struggling with being overweight and multiple health issues when she was given a chance to attend one of my training institutes. On her drive across Iowa, she started second-guessing herself.

"Halfway there, I decided to turn off the interstate and go back," she shared, "but when I got to the next exit it was closed. I knew that was a sign, and I forced myself to take one of the biggest risks of my life. I'm so grateful I did. It changed everything."

Each small risk, such as talking to a stranger while waiting in line, or asking for help from a friend, strengthens our risk muscle to be ready for those golden opportunities that show up when we least expect them.

Krissy was, as we all are at times, afraid of *failure*. At the training we helped her redefine that word.

What is Failure?

- *Failure is merely Feedback.*
- *Failure is Delay, not Defeat.*
- *Failure is a Bruise, not a Tattoo.*

As you travel these 8 High-Ways, you'll discover that the road to success is never a straight line, not even for the most dedicated of Ideals. Your road to success with the program will be full of setbacks and surprises. Accept and embrace that there will be detours, delays, and sharp turns. The important thing to realize is this:

> *Practice doesn't make perfect.*
> *It makes progress.*

Stay the course and each week I guarantee you will have a Release or a Realization. Neither are failures. Both are successes and worth celebrating!

Once Krissy could see failure in a new light, she was ready to see risk in a new light.

What is Risk?

We have been taught that:

- *Risks are dangerous*
- *Risks are irresponsible*
- *Risks are bad*

Unfortunately, those who taught us the negative perspective of risk were most likely living in fear of failure themselves.

When you ask those you admire the most - those who you see as living a truly happy and healthy life - you will find that they see risk-taking completely differently. Risks are **risky**, yes, but they are a necessity for a fully actualized life, and they are very, very **good**.

At a turning point in my recovery from a life of fear and low self-esteem, I redefined Risk as:

> *Run To, Not From.*

In **8 to Your IdealWeight**, there is no such thing as a negative risk because:

> Risk = Run To   Escape = Run From

A Run to is a positive thing.

Ask yourself:

- *Was joining this program Running to or Running from?*
- *Is overeating to comfort myself Running to or Running from?*
- *Is hiding my thoughts and feelings from those closest to me Running to or Running from?*
- *Is asking someone to be my Gratitude Partner Running to or Running from?*

Once you have a clear definition of risk, it becomes clear that you're either moving toward or away from your dreams. It will be just as clear that *not* risking is much more "dangerous" to our well-being.

"Avoiding danger is no safer in the long run than outright exposure. Life is either a daring adventure or nothing."

- Helen Keller

How to Make Every Decision and Know It's the Right One for You

Fear of an uncertain future can stop us from doing great things, and can keep us holding onto things that hurt us. For example, you might be holding onto clutter for reasons of comfort and security, even if the clutter gives you anxiety and costs you a lot of money to store. Or maybe you're staying in a job you don't like because you're afraid of taking the plunge and failing.

It turns out there is a simple **Formula for Decision Making** that works every time when you're making a decision. Simply ask yourself:

If I had no fear, what would I do?

Of course we all have fears, but we can use our imagination. If I had no fear, what would I do? What would I stop doing? Where would I go? Who would I be?

"I want to meet some new friends, but I've always been terribly shy," I heard from an Ideal who had just moved to a larger city. I reminded her that shy is a decision, not a disease.

As it turns out, researchers tell us that taking big risks, like dreaming big dreams, feels as good (creates as many endorphins) as **falling in love**. Talk about 95'ing! That's a really high high!

The Myth of Sitting Still

I recall a day when my daughter came home from 3rd grade all excited. "Mom, we found out today how you can tell if a plant is alive!"

"How Sweetheart?"

"If it's growing!"

That's how we can tell if a person is alive. There is no sitting still on the Power Pyramid of life. To "sit still" in life is actually to regress because it requires digging in our heels against what is. Life around us and within us is always changing.

Did you "sit still" when the latest cell phones came out or did you learn the new technology? Did you use the same parenting skills with your child when they were 14 as you did when they were 4? Of course not. Sitting still means falling further and further behind, and soon we will be at odds with life.

We don't have to fall in love with change to be successful, but we do have to make friends with it. When we learn to "grow with the flow," we see that it can take us where we want to go - toward our biggest dreams.

You are making dozens of changes in how you think, how you eat, and what you say to yourself when you look in the mirror. Congratulations! Your risks will yield rewards.

> *"Your life doesn't get better by chance.*
> *It gets better by change."*

> - Jim Rohn

The 3 Levels of Risk

When Ideals let me know they're "just not a risk taker," I ask them to look again. In this world there is no other kind of being. But some of us started off as big risk takers when we were children and have slowly weakened our risk taker muscles. So let's go to the risk gym and get back in shape!

Look over the Risk lists on the following pages and ask yourself these 3 questions:

- *What 5 risks have you already taken? Pat yourself on the back!*

- *What are 5 smaller risks you could set as goals over the next few weeks?*

- *What are 5 larger risks you could set as dreams over the next year?*

Beginning Risks:

- *Say No to free food*
- *Go to bed earlier*
- *Ask for what you really want at a restaurant*
- *Get a massage*
- *Stop watching the news*
- *Wear brightly colored prints and solids**
- *Color your hair*
- *Talk to a stranger in an elevator or on an airplane*
- *Go ice skating or rollerskating*
- *Volunteer at a shelter*
- *Go dancing or join a Zumba class*
- *Sell something on Craigslist*
- *Sing in the shower*
- *Go canoeing or paddleboating or snorkeling*
- *Take (healthy) food to a neighbor or someone who's hurting*
- *Journal*
- *Make a Dream Board*
- *Call a creditor and work out payments on your bills*
- *Get your picture taken in a photo booth*
- *Make a private YouTube video*
- *Take a class in cooking, dancing, sewing, a foreign language, sign language, painting, piano, archery, shooting, horseback riding, tennis, pickleball, aromatherapy, magic, communication, debt release (Dave Ramsey has a great one)*
- *Join a choir*
- *Tell or text someone your weight*

- *Ask someone to be your walking partner/gratitude partner*
- *Donate blood*
- *Travel to a larger city or visit a farm*
- *Eat at a new vegetarian or ethnic restaurant*
- *Learn to play Bridge or Mah Jongg*

From one Ideal:

"I have chosen to accept myself in my body regardless of my size and love wearing beautiful bright colors. There are so many women who tell me they wish they could wear the bright prints I do, but it's just because they tell themselves they can't that they don't. If you believe you can, so will everyone else!"

- Barb F.

Intermediate Risks:

- *Invite a new friend to go to a movie*
- *Look for a new job*
- *Get on a dating site*
- *Buy or sell a car*
- *Go on a cruise*
- *Learn to water ski, snow ski, kayak, or sail*
- *Join a yoga, tai chi or meditation class*
- *Wear shorts or a swimsuit in public*
- *Go on a solo or couple's retreat*
- *Walk out of a movie you find offensive*
- *Ask your boss for a raise or share an idea with him/her*
- *Go to a church other than your own*
- *Write a letter to the editor or call into a radio show*
- *Join Toastmasters*

- *Start your own private Facebook group page*
- *Go on Meetup.com and join a group of like-minded folks*
- *Play laser tag or paintball*
- *Invest in the stock market*
- *Make a Youtube.com video and share it with the public*
- *Audition for a play*
- *Hike up a mountain*
- *Go ziplining, parasailing, or whitewater rafting*
- *Write your spouse a love letter*
- *Start a Bible study/book club*
- *Admit you were wrong about something without excuses*
- *Wear a little black (or red) dress in public*
- *Have your aura picture taken*
- *Give your first public talk*
- *Contact someone you haven't talked to for years*

Advanced Risks:

(Note: Each one of these risks has been taken by an Ideal!)

- *Write a book*
- *Sell one of your art pieces for the first time*
- *Start a new business*
- *Move to a new city*
- *Get married*
- *Buy or sell a home*
- *Find a Coach or Counselor and make an appointment*

- Learn to ride a motorcycle or fly a plane
- Learn to hunt mountain lions
- Go skydiving, surfing, scuba diving or rock climbing
- Enter a speaking contest
- Travel abroad
- Tell someone you are in love with them before they tell you
- Run for office
- Send your book off to an agent or publisher
- Record one of your songs and share it on cdbaby.com
- Go hot air ballooning
- Tell a secret you've been hiding for months or years
- Leave an abusive situation
- Go back to school and get an advanced degree
- Get certified as a scuba instructor/yoga instructor/massage therapist/8 to Your IdealWeight Coach

I recently had an Ideal who was concerned about some women at her church talking behind her back. In my letter, I wrote:

In this world there are two kinds of people: Those who talk about other people, and those who are talked about because their lives are so interesting. Which would you rather be? You've got this.

20 Seconds

Have you seen the movie, *"We Bought a Zoo"*? It's based on a true story and I highly recommend it. One of my all-time favorite quotes came from that film:

"Sometimes all you need is 20 seconds of insane courage. Just, literally, 20 seconds of embarrassing bravery. And I promise you, something great will come of it."

– from *"We Bought a Zoo"*

Sometimes a risk that might look small to someone else is huge to us. I remember the day my first book came out. I didn't want to go out of the house for fear it was a flop. Taking a risk by sharing our hearts and our truth takes great courage. Here is a beautiful example of an Ideal who exemplified that courage.

Brenda's Risk

One of my favorite examples of risk comes from an Ideal who emailed me asking about the class.

Brenda was in her early 40's when we met. Her voice was so faint on our first phone call, I could barely hear what she was saying. I told her that I would be asking some questions to see if joining my small group felt like a fit to both of us. At the end of the conversation, when I invited her in, I heard tears in her voice as she thanked me for accepting her into the program.

What I did not learn until later was that at that time Brenda's self-esteem was so low she often didn't want to get out of bed. Although she had been seeing a counselor and a psychiatrist, she had been feeling hopeless and stuck for a long time. That changed once she joined the program. Even the counselor and her physician were amazed at the changes in her.

After her 30-pound release, she became an IdealWeight Coach, and wrote on her Facebook page...

"God has truly blessed me with this awesome journey over the past 6 months...one that I will continue on for the rest of my life! My entire life and body have been transformed in the most positive ways. I am beyond grateful, and it is my intention to carry this amazing lightness into the world, and share this wonderful gift with others!"

- Brenda F.

As Brenda reminds us:

No risks = no rewards. Big risks = big rewards.

"Do one thing every day that scares you."

- Eleanor Roosevelt

Setting Boundaries and Saying No

Risking isn't just about doing things we've never done. It can also include the decision to stop doing things we've always done. And that means making friends with the word "No."

Without No in your vocabulary, your Yes means nothing.

Think about it. We have all known people (perhaps ourselves) who "couldn't" say No. We learned not to trust those people, because we never knew if their Yes meant Yes, No, or Maybe.

I have met new Ideals who had been making everyone else's crises their own and paying a high price. I have loved seeing them learn to stand up for themselves, set boundaries, and create a life of balance and peace.

If you feel guilty about saying No, do this check:

There is such a thing as healthy guilt. When we step outside of our moral boundaries, it's healthy to feel a discomfort or guilt about our actions. However, when we are within those boundaries, and allow another person's opinions to make us feel guilty, it is not healthy.

Healthy Guilt/Discomfort - behaviors (actions) outside our moral guidelines

Unhealthy Guilt/Discomfort - behaviors (actions) within our moral guidelines

A "No-ing" Worth Celebrating

One Ideal had a mother who fed her children so much sugar when she had them over that they came home with stomach aches and headaches each time. Another Ideal was asked by her daughter to drive the kids to and from school every day "now that she was retired." A third Ideal was asked to take money out of her family's savings to buy the family home so it could be kept in the family when Mom and Dad left, even though she and her spouse already had plans for the savings.

Each of these Ideals found the courage to risk saying "No," and as a result, did not need to turn to sugar for comfort. They felt comforted in knowing they had cared for themselves in a very loving way.

In my early recovery from endless people pleasing, the behavior of saying No was so foreign to me, I had to ease into it slowly. At first, I couldn't say No, so I just didn't say Yes. While it was a start, I eventually learned to say No without guilt.

In the following list of ways to say No, some are beginner steps, while others are more assertive and take greater courage. Which one is closest to your current communication style? Which one would you like to utilize?

10 Ways to Say No

1) **Avoid people and places that are uncomfortable entirely.** This is a temporary solution at best. Build up your courage and backbone so that you aren't giving away your power and running from the people in your life.

2) **Break physical contact or phone contact once a boundary crossing occurs.** You can walk away (to the restroom), hang up ("There's someone at the door, I need to go") or just say you're tired and need to lay down.

3) **Use someone else as an excuse, such as,** "My parents/ husband wouldn't be comfortable with that, so no thanks."

4) **Delay your answer.** Consider using a phrase like "I'll consider that in the future, but right now, no," or "Let me think about it. I'm not sure right now. "

5) **Be vague, such as,** "I'm not in a situation right now where I can say yes," or "for personal reasons I can't take that on right now."

6) **Offer an alternative.** "You won't be able to bring your new boyfriend to our dinner party because we're full to the

brim, but we'd love to meet him. Maybe we could go out to dinner the following week."

7) **Say you're busy.** "I've got something going that evening, sorry." (It could be a hot bath!)

8) **Use the broken record technique and just keep repeating "No thanks."**

9) **Change the subject.** "No thanks. That a new haircut?"

Once you have mastered these early levels, you are ready for one of the most assertive responses:

10) **"No, I won't be doing that, but thank you for asking."**

Notice, with this last reply you are not giving them a reason why you're saying No because then they'll likely argue about the reason. When we are most assertive, we do not need to defend our decisions. We simply state them.

> *"You cannot live a brave life without disappointing some people."*
>
> - Oprah Winfrey

 Heartwork for High-Way 2

1. Ask for what you want in new ways this week, even if it's "dressing on the side" for your salad at a restaurant.

2. Risk asking three people this week one or both of these questions:

1. What is one of your dreams?

2. If you had no fear, what would you do?
(Be prepared to be asked in return!)

3. For the Mirror Mantra this week, use words like "brave" and "confident" and "a risk-taker" for affirmation #3.

 Partner/Reflection Questions

For your sharing with your partner this week, consider discussing the following:

1. What are 2-3 risks I've taken since picking up this book?

2. If I had no fear, what would I do? What would I stop doing? Where would I go? Who would I be?

3. Where is it time to say "no" and set boundaries in my life? What support could I ask for in that process?

4. Share some risks you'd like to take from the 3 Levels in this chapter. What risk could you commit to taking this coming week? This month?

HIGH-WAY 3:
FULL RESPONSIBILITY

"Our deepest fear is not that we are powerless. Our deepest fear is that we are powerful beyond measure."

– Marianne Williamson,
author of *"A Return to Love"*

Defining Full Responsibility

In *8 to Great* I defined Full Responsibility this way:

Full Responsibility is moving from B.C. to A.D.: from Blaming and Complaining to Acting and Dreaming.

When we B.C. (Blame and Complain), we are giving our power away to the situations or individuals involved. We are, in essence, saying, "If only he/she they would...then I could be happy."

Instead, we can A.D., choosing to Act (such as getting on a Get Real program like you did) and Dream (such as creating a Dream Board as we did in High-Way 1).

We have a choice in every moment, and the happiest among us remember never to put the key to our happiness in someone else's pocket.

The Key to Your Freedom

The desire to be free is universal. Whether it's our desire to be 'free of,' or the desire to be 'free to,' we all long for greater freedom.

Then the day comes when we realize we have had it all along. And that we have given away much of it, unknowingly. We do it every time we say, "I'll be happy when..." and then wait for "when" to arrive.

Do you recognize any of these "I'll be happy when" excuses?

- *When I find someone to love me (giving your relationship status your power)*
- *When my son gets a job (giving your son your power)*
- *When my co-workers respect me (giving your co-workers your power)*
- *When I release these next 10-50 pounds (giving the scale your power)*
- *When I no longer am worried about my mother falling (It's not in your control. Is she ready for a nursing facility?)*

   "It's not your job to like me - it's mine."

- Byron Katie,
author of *"The Work"*

One of the attributes of those who have found long-lasting peace and joy is that instead of waiting for people or circumstances to change in order to be happy, they find their happy place each day by choosing their focus. As their focus changes, their situations change as well.

Taking Our Power Back from the Scale

The scale can only give you a numerical reflection of
your relationship with gravity. It cannot measure your
compassion, talent, beauty, purpose, possibilities,
courage or love.

No matter what bumps life throws in our path, we can always
find a better-feeling thought to focus on. It could be as
simple as finding three new gratitudes.

I have seen Ideals who've plateaued, or even gained at the
end of a week. Yet instead of becoming discouraged at the
temporary setback (often caused by a menstrual cycle), they
took their eyes off the scale numbers and made lists of the
other benefits they were grateful to receive through this
program. One Ideal's list included these:

Since starting this program:

- *I routinely ask for what I want.*
- *I have more confidence.*
- *I get up early to walk.*
- *I am feeding my body healthy, whole foods.*
- *I recognize my emotional eating patterns.*
- *I catch and release my "worry thoughts" more quickly.*
- *I don't feel guilty about taking time for me.*
- *I am excited to find things to release each day.*

Knowing that feeling better is just a thought away gives us not
only great power, but great responsibility. Full Responsibility

is acknowledging that we are not victims, because in every moment, we have the freedom and power to choose.

Alaina was a great example of Risk and Full Responsibility in sharing her poem on this topic:

Dear MK,

My name is Alaina Browning. I live in a remote area in Montana. I am a rancher and Wildland firefighter and have six daughters. On the 8 to Your IdealWeight Program I have released 40 pounds. I've always dreamed of being published and love writing stories and poems. I wrote a poem two months ago and it has taken me this long to get up the courage to take this risk! It is a dream of mine to publish a story or poem in a book. I wrote this poem for my fellow Ideals when they were struggling. They loved it and encouraged me to share it with you. So here it goes:

SCALE

Scale you do not define me
You're just a gauging tool
When you do not move
I will not let you make me your fool

You cannot measure happiness
You cannot give a hug
You're just a decoration
Like the bathroom rug

Your number is not who I am
I know I'm so much more
You cannot measure the hopes and dreams
That I have in store

Ideals,
Time is a gift we are given every day
But life is too short to give our power away

No matter what the number
Remember to just grin
Our beauty is not external
Our beauty comes from within

- Alaina Browning 4-10-16

The Day I Found My Voice

I am in charge of my life.
I'm not in charge of yours.

We are not responsible for how other people respond to us. When we tie ourselves into knots and withhold self-loving behaviors to avoid the possibility of upsetting others, we are giving away our power. I know the danger of people pleasing all too well.

After completing my month in the shelter, my dear family, in shock at hearing of my situation, drove hours to visit me in

Omaha. I still recall when we were sitting around the table at the Chinese restaurant that first evening. As the meal was served in small metal covered serving dishes, we passed them around the table.

As I was dishing out rice from the third platter onto my plate, my mother spoke up from two chairs down. "Honey, the rice goes underneath the vegetables." In that moment something in me shifted.

"If we all focus on our own meals this evening, it will probably feel a lot better," I said quietly.

My family all stopped eating and looked up to see her reaction. After a stunned moment of silence, she stood so quickly that her chair tipped back and she said in a loud voice, "You used to be such fun to be around!" She then headed off to the women's bathroom.

"You may all continue eating," I told the remaining family members. "I'm not going after her."

Mom returned to the table five minutes later, yet didn't speak to me for the next few hours. I was sad and very scared. Was this the price I had to pay to live the truths I had learned and take responsibility for my life? Was I required to sacrifice my relationship with my beloved Mom?

Later that evening, she walked up to me and hugged me. It marked a new phase of mutual respect in our relationship, and eventually led to her finding her voice in her marriage to my father. Today she is very good at asking for what she wants.

It takes courage to take charge of your own life. It also takes courage to release charge over another's, as we hear in this version of the AA Serenity Prayer:

God, grant me the serenity to accept the things I cannot change - others;
the courage to change the things I can - myself;
And the wisdom to know the difference.

Is it a Should or a Want?

One of the phrases that helped me heal from my people pleasing was this one:

Don't should on yourself, and don't should on other people.

"Shoulds" are those thoughts we carry around inside of us that originate from other people. The next time you hear yourself "shoulding" on yourself, even if it's just mentally, stop and ask yourself, do I want to do that? If the answer is "No," then ask yourself if the task can be delayed, delegated or eliminated without causing any real harm.

Another simple way to avoid the judgment of shoulds is to replace "I should" with "I could."

Ideal Examples

Jeanette shared that the replacement phrase was helpful for her:

"Before this IdealWeight program I was a total 'shoulder.' I would 'should' on myself 100 times a day. Now I can recognize what this does to my attitude, and so can my husband. Together we're moving from 'should' to 'could.'"

Bobbi recognized her pattern of taking better care of others than she was of herself, but wasn't sure how to make the shift. Her wake-up call came with a visit from her sister.

"At first when my sister would visit, I would find myself believing I "should" buy all sorts of off-program snacks for her which she would never eat. Then who would be left to consume them? Now when my sister visits, I ask her to bring her own snacks. She doesn't mind at all!"

Rene was always giving and doing for her family. When her daughter had her first child, she shared, "Between my full-time job and my volunteering for church, I had a full life before the baby. Now my daughter expects me to watch the baby every evening. I feel like I should, but I can hardly see straight I'm so exhausted."

After we talked, she decided to make up a calendar with two times each week she could go over and to share it with her daughter. Then, when asked to run errands or do the laundry, she could say that she'd gladly take care of those items at that time.

According to Rene, questioning her "should" restored her energy levels. When she and her daughter knew where the boundaries were, they both felt calmer.

The Gift of Intuition

When we release trying to be who the world says we "should" be, we relax and are free to be who we are. This opens our hearts to hear the voice of our intuition. Intuition is that inner feminine gift (that men have also) of receiving insights that go against the logical and rational.

Looking back over my life, many, if not most, of my best decisions defied logic. I simply was listening to the "wants" of my heart rather than the "shoulds" of my mind. Sometimes it was as simple as taking another route, unaware that a bridge was closed that would have prevented my on-time arrival. Sometimes it's much bigger.

At 55 years old, my friends asked me why I was moving from my home of 30 years to live in Kansas City, where I knew almost no one. Since I had no logical reasons, my answer was simply, "Why not?"

Today it is crystal clear to those who know me well that it was there in Dorothy's Kansas that my joy journey awaited me.

"Told you so."

Sincerely,
Your Intuition

Favors vs. Gifts

Full Responsibility includes staying in balance. I have seen so many Ideals over-care for others, at the expense of under-caring for themselves. So it would serve us to look at when giving and doing is healthy, and when it is unhealthy.

A simple way to distinguish them is to look at the difference between a Gift and a Favor.

F.A.V.O.R. = Feeling Acceptable and Valuable Only when Rescuing

Years ago, I discerned that the differences between a Gift and a Favor included:

A Gift:

- *It's a want, not a should.*
- *You won't feel guilty if you don't give it.*
- *It's coming from your surplus.*

A Favor:

- *It's a should, not a want.*
- *They ask you (often silently) to "trust them" when they haven't built up enough "cash" in your relationship account. There is no emotional collateral, like an unsecured loan.*
- *You feel guilty when you consider saying no because you do have the resources (some money/ a working car/ an extra bedroom, etc.)*
- *You will pay a high price for fulfilling their request that will put you in the red as far as time, money, or energy.*

Question: If you had a bankrupt friend, who kept making terrible investments and then came to you each month to pay their rent, would it be healthy or loving to keep giving them rent money?

Of course not. So why, when someone gets themselves into a crisis life situation with a bad relationship, a bad car decision, etc. do we sometimes feel that we are responsible for rescuing them just because we have something they don't?

"In the Bible we read, 'Whatsoever you do to the least of my brethren,' but what if the least of my brethren is me?"

- Carl Jung

When you see where this is happening in your life, instead of saying Yes to a "should" favor request, consider using a phrase like this one:

"No, I won't be able to do that for too many reasons to explain, but thank you for asking."

Over-giving and endless favors are part of an out-of-balance life that can send us back into our addictive behaviors. Jill's situation was one example...

"My new co-worker is sleeping in her car because she's going through a divorce," Jill shared with me during a coaching session. "She doesn't get paid for another week and I have an extra bedroom, so I'm thinking of inviting her to stay with me. I want to know your thoughts."

I shared that I was seeing a pattern in her life. "Jill, you remind me of the old me, the woman who was addicted to being 'nice.' As your coach I am inviting you to abstain from doing favors like this for one month. Let's focus on getting your finances and your health back. There are shelters that woman can go to."

"That feels kind of selfish," she replied honestly. "But I trust you, so I'll give it a try."

The following day when her new co-worker didn't show up for work, someone thought to check the police report. She had been picked up on drug charges. Jill had averted a crisis.

"One of the most shocking findings of my research was that the most compassionate people I interviewed were also those with the clearest boundaries."

- Brene Brown

The Power of Letting Go

One of my favorite poems about Full Responsibility is an anonymous one.

Letting Go

To "let go" does not mean to stop caring,
it means I can't do it for someone else.

To "let go" is not to cut myself off,
it's the realization I can't control another.

To "let go" is not to enable,
but to allow learning from natural consequences.

To "let go" is to admit powerlessness,
which means the outcome is not in my hands,
only my attitude is.

To "let go" is not to try to change or blame another,
it's to make the most of myself.

To "let go" is not to care for,
but to care about.

To "let go" is not to fix,
but to be supportive.

To "let go" is not to judge,
but to allow another to be a human being.

To "let go" is not to deny,
but to accept.

To "let go" is not to nag, scold or argue,
but instead to search out my own shortcomings and
correct them.

To "let go" is not to criticize and regulate anybody,
but to try to become what I dream I can be.

To "let go" is not to regret the past,
but to be grateful for the present and have hope for
the future.

To "let go" is to fear less,
and love more.

Letting Go of Our Stuff

When I started my first **8 to Your IdealWeight** support group with 10 women, I knew I wanted the program to be more than just about releasing weight. I had a hunch that, like me, each of those women was holding onto old "stuff" that drained their energy and weighed them down.

As I'd guessed, one of my coaching clients had multiple properties and "couldn't move until she sold them." Another single woman had an elderly mother whom she called or checked on daily, so that even after her retirement, she was feeling chained to her small hometown.

A third had three houses of items crammed into one house and garage, and used "not having the time to clean them out" as her reason for not following her dream of moving to Phoenix.

Whether we have a lot of physical weight or physical stuff to release, it can't be done in a day. That was why I decided to make one of the daily check-ins with my clients the 4th F: Freedom: **Did you release something today?**

The results have been astounding and consistent. Whether it's a garbage sack full or a van full of "no-longer-neededs," the response from the releaser is always the same, "I feel so much lighter!"

Looking over my overly-full closet one day, I made myself a promise. Either I would wear each item during that month or I would give it away. My trips to Salvation Army that month were frequent and freeing!

You may also discover that you're hanging onto things for others. "But what if my kids want all these pictures of their childhood?" we wonder. When I asked mine what they wanted instead of assuming, I found they did not want any photos other than the ones they already had. The last thing I threw out before my move to Florida was 23 scrapbooks full of pictures. It felt great.

(Yes, for those of you hyperventilating right now, I kept four of them for me!)

Let your lighter shine!

Bonita was one of those who shared that with each bag of release she felt lighter. In her words, *"After releasing nearly 60 pounds of excess weight and likely 500 pounds of excess stuff, I am thrilled with who I am today. Thanks to this process I am more confident, live with greater clarity and am more true to myself. If someone offered me a million dollars to regain the weight and go back to who I was, I'd say 'No Way!' What I have now is priceless!"*

Now that's what freedom feels like.

What is More Important than My Feeling Good?

Full Responsibility is refusing to make excuses. Excuses like, "I was traveling" or "We're so busy at work" are just exit signs. They indicate that you've taken your eye off the prize. Where do you want to be in six months or a year? Who do you want to be? Remember...

If it is to be, it is up to me.

Life happens. If you are experiencing a sudden illness of a loved one, or even a death, be easy on yourself. Take time off from any concerns about food. But if the stressors are the usual ones, it's time to ask yourself some hard questions.

Which of the following have I been making more important than reaching my IdealWeight?

- *Fitting in with friends at a neighborhood or work party*
- *Reassuring my mother-in-law/mother/friend that she is a good cook*
- *My kids learning to eat healthy with me right now*
- *Volunteering for nonprofit organizations*
- *Growing my business faster*
- *Having a spotlessly clean home*
- *Not letting people know I'm changing my eating habits*
- *Saving money (indicates a misunderstanding of the program foods)*
- *Staying up late to talk to my spouse/partner/teen*
- *Keeping my pain a secret*
- *Having a few drinks to unwind on the weekends*
- *Working overtime and not setting limits on my workload*

If you selected any of the above, it may be time to write yourself a letter recommitting to your promises, or reread the Personal Agreement that you wrote when you began this course.

I Could Stay on the Program If Only...

From the list below, select which issue is your biggest trigger these days, then move from B.C. to A.D. by taking action:

I'm angry so I eat - Change something. Ask for what you want. Set a boundary with "No, I won't be doing that, but thank you for asking." Eat a gluten free cracker or talk to your **Ideal** Partner or your coach.

I'm lonely/bored so I eat - Join www.meetup.com. Volunteer. Watch inspiring TED talks. Learn sign language. Get a pet. Take a class. Teach a community college class. Talk to your **Ideal** Partner or your coach or a counselor.

I'm stressed about money so I eat - Remember that when you take control of this *one* thing you'll be able to take care of the next thing (money). In addition, you'll feel better about applying for (and getting) a better paying job at your IdealWeight. Talk to your **Ideal** Partner or your coach.

I'm depressed so I watch TV and I eat - Buy a romance novel. (My latest favorite is "Big Girl Panties" by Stephanie Evanovich.) Limit your TV hours or cancel cable. Talk to your **Ideal** Partner or your coach or a counselor.

It's too tiring to cook two meals - Have your spouse/partner/teenager cook. Hire a cook. Give the kids KFC every night for 8 weeks. Buy a rotisserie chicken and pre-cooked veggies at the grocery store deli. Join a service that helps you pre-cook meals. Talk to your **Ideal** Partner or your coach.

How High-Way 3 Changed Her Life

Teresa's Story

I guess it would be safe to say that a thermometer has a job and that a thermostat has a job. A thermometer takes the temperature of the room, while the thermostat sets the temperature of the room.

I found myself in MK's class years ago and we were coasting along just fine until she came up with this phrase "In 8 to Great we don't believe in adult victims."

At that point I immediately shut down and it was like "wham" for me. I remember thinking, "Okay, this is not what I signed up for." It was the worst news I had ever heard.

It was the worst news because it meant that I was responsible for everything that was going on in my life, and that was one place I did not want to go. The only reason I didn't walk out was because there were so many people packed into that room and I didn't want to bring attention to myself. So I sat there.

As she continued to talk, I was soon able to understand that if I was the problem, I was the solution. That was the most powerful moment of my life.

I realized from that moment on that if I could cause all of this havoc and problems in my life then I could also be the one to cause all these amazing things to happen. I decided that I would forever be the thermostat when I walked into the room. That I would be this bright light, and the worst thing that could happen is I could just be a bright light among other bright lights. I was going to call the shots in my life from that day forward. It was a life-changing moment.

- Teresa R. Getman,
8 to Great Master Trainer

"The truth will set you free,
but first it will make you miserable."

- Rev. Sky St. John

Taking Our Power Back from Binges

The Beliefs Behind Binging

After two decades of teaching *8 to Great* to recovering alcoholics, I learned that an addict's binges are never brought on by one event, such as a poor job evaluation or the loss of a loved one. They are the cumulative result of giving one's power away to heavy thoughts hundreds of times throughout a week, a month or a year. The trigger event is simply the "last straw."

Believing that we are victims is the heaviest belief of all. We can start to feel powerless to make real change.

Yet, as adults, we are never victims. Our recovery requires us to start noticing the people and events where we give our power away. Once we recognize the triggers, the next time a painful experience shows up, it's easier to catch our heavy, negative (fear and judgment) thoughts and return our focus to those that feel lighter.

The Heaviness of Fear

I recall one Ideal who couldn't figure out why she was overeating at buffets and accepting food that wasn't on her program from friends and family members. As we talked, we discovered that "free" food was her trigger. When I asked if she was facing money issues, she shared that she was worried about her cash flow due to being out of work from an injury.

Her extremely heavy fear was that she would run out of money if she didn't take the "free" food. Once we added up the cost of hanging onto her extra weight and of the health problems it was bringing her, she reframed her thoughts about "free" food as extremely expensive, and released 20 pounds during her first 8-week course!

You hold the key. When you become **aware of your triggers and acknowledge your power over them**, you are back on track. When you accept Full Responsibility for your life, you are free!

Tools for Ending the Binging Cycle

You now have the tools to end your binging cycles.

First, like an alcoholic who finds they cannot drink without excess, you're becoming more aware of sugar's effect on your appetite, allowing you to choose foods that decrease cravings rather than increase them.

Second, you're becoming more aware of your thoughts, so that you can choose which ones you "feed." There is always a version of a heavy thought that feels better. An example would be reframing, "I failed today," to "I discovered one of my triggers today. I'm grateful to know that I can ask for help."

Another example might be moving from "I'll show them" as an excuse to go off program to: "They have no right to treat me that way. It's absolutely valid that I'm really upset about it. There is no way I'm giving them and their actions the power to pull me off my program!"

To review, to prevent binges:

1. *Take charge of your sugar intake*
2. *Take charge of your thought focus*

Life is My Mirror

In **8 to Your IdealWeight**, part of our healing is making friends with the mirrors we have detested in the past.

Getting angry at a mirror for what it tells us is missing the gift it offers. Mirrors are our friends, and as we move into greater self-awareness, we start to see reflections all around us. Which of them are you ready to see?

- *What if the regret and guilt you're carrying within you is reflected in the piles of old and unused items surrounding you in your home?*
- *What if how worthy of respect you feel is reflected in how much others respect you at home and work?*

Life is our mirror.

What is Eating You?

What if that individual who frustrates you the most in your life is one of your best mirrors, and has one of the greatest gifts to give you? It could be the "negative" co-worker that grates you with their endless complaints, or that stranger that honked at you unnecessarily.

Frustrations can be seen as growth opportunities when we see that the enemy is "in-a-me."

The next time you're frustrated with someone, ask yourself: **"What about them reminds me of what frustrates me about myself?"**

Awhile back I was listening to a speaker who began with the statement, "Alright, no questions or comments during my talk. I'll take questions at the end but I don't want you to throw me off." Well that comment threw me off, because as a speaker myself I like to engage with my audience members, and as an audience member, I like to engage.

If I started a little triggered, by the end of the hour I was absolutely agitated. After the talk I jumped up from my chair and went for a walk to ask myself, **"What about him reminds me of what frustrates me about myself?"**

The first word that came to me was "boring." I didn't think he connected with his audience. I knew that judging a person does not define who they are. It defines who we are, so I turned it around and asked, "What is it about him being boring that reminds me of what frustrates me about myself?"

My light bulbs flashed. "Of course! I hate to be boring. It's something I would rather die than be." As a public speaker certainly, but even at a dinner party, I always do my best not to be the "B" word.

So, what was the cure for my discomfort? The deepest cure of all: **unconditional self-love.**

As I walked, I said aloud, "MK, here's the deal. Sometimes you're boring. But you know what? You're lovable even when you're boring." It felt weird at first, but I said it many times over and it got easier and easier, "MK, even when you're boring, and sometimes you are, you're still very lovable."

Not only did my peaceful spirit return, but my memory of his presentation is filled with nothing but gratitude. I felt great appreciation for the lesson learned from my 'perfect' teacher. He had helped me get back to a more unconditional love of myself.

You spot it, you got it.

I've had many Ideals complain that people are rude to those who are overweight. Whenever we're upset with how we're being treated, who needs to change first? We do. This mirror called Life will always reflect how we think about and treat ourselves. When we take Full Responsibility, the best news and the hardest news is that the only person we need to change is ourselves.

 Heartwork for High-Way 3

1. With what people in your life are you ready to find your voice? Write out a letter you might send to them, but rather than send it, learn from it and burn it.

2. Look ahead to the coming week. Do you have some "should" activities that could be delegated or eliminated? If not, can you change them to a "want?" (Because you appreciate your paycheck, for example?)

3. Answer these questions in your journal:

> What has triggered my binges in the past?
> What new awareness do I have now to end that cycle?

4. What quality in others has been triggering you lately? Where do you see that quality in yourself? Can you love yourself in spite of having that flaw?

5. When you are ready for the world to fall more in love with you, write yourself a love letter. Keep it in a special place to read from time to time.

"Things do not change, we change."

- Henry David Thoreau

 Partner/Reflection Questions

For your sharing this week, consider discussing the following:

- *Are there some boundaries I am ready to set and communicate?*

- *Are there some "shoulds" I am ready to delegate or eliminate?*

- *Am I willing to take the "No Favors Challenge" for a day? A week? The rest of the 8-week program?*

- *If you're still feeling tempted by sugary foods, take time to journal a dialogue between the part of you that really wants to release your extra weight and the part of you that still wants to eat what you've always eaten. Make sure they both get equal time. What you write will come from your subconscious and will often amaze you. When finished, take the risk and share it with your Partner or Coach.*

No secrets = No regrets.

HIGH-WAY 4: FEEL ALL YOUR FEELINGS

The Real Reason We Overeat

"The need to hang onto extra weight is caused by a perceived need for protection, running from our feelings, and self-rejection."

– Louise Hay,
author of *"You Can Heal Your Life"*

It can feel empowering to know there's one primary and personal reason why we overeat, and that it has nothing to do with willpower or genetics. The reason is the same as it is for all addictions:

We overeat so that we don't have to feel.

Life is all about feelings. Some emotions feel better than others. The problems arise only when we try to hide from or outrun those that are painful. They will always catch up with us.

Sometimes people misinterpret what I do as a motivational speaker. "Can you help me to be happier?" they ask. I reply that the answer depends on if they are willing to also feel their sadness and anger. We only have one heart, and it is either open or closed. When it's open, it feels more pain as well as more pleasure. If you're truly willing to open your heart to the magnificent feeling of being fully alive, this High-Way can help.

Emotion comes from the words "Energy in Motion." Think of trying to stop the rain or the wind. It would only make you exhausted, which is why, when we try to suppress our feelings, we are tired all the time. It's also why, when we start to allow our feelings again, we feel energized, often as though we have a new lease on life.

It's time we learn to honor and embrace our feelings, seeing them as a necessary and healthy part of being human. Like the weather, our feelings are always changing, so seeing them as temporary is a good first step. It also helps to remember that pain is part of every human journey, but it doesn't have to be our enemy. It can make us bitter or better. It is our choice.

**Pain is a required part of the human condition.
Suffering is optional.**

One Ideal shared, "Now that I know that my pain is not 'special,' and that everyone has hidden wounds, I am ready to deal with it." She had learned not to shoot the second arrow.

Anger can't define us. Sadness can't make us sick. But our reactions to them can. There is a Buddhist teaching that refers to the painful event as "the first arrow." It teaches that the first arrow is not the dangerous one. It is the second arrow, our reaction, that causes suffering.

Tanya's Story of Her "Very Hard Day"

Tanya had signed up for weekly phone calls with me during her 8-week program, and I loved talking with her. She was dedicated to the process and making huge changes in her life while she watched her teenager benefit from her new eating habits as well.

But one day, four weeks in, she shared that she had had "a very hard day." She then went into how, at a recent church event, she was able to pass up mashed potatoes and gravy, only to decide to have dessert.

In her mind the problem was the food. My coaching experience told me otherwise.

"I'd like you to do some journaling," I began. "Write about what circumstances might have worn you down before you went to that event. Why were you more vulnerable that day? Was it fatigue? A new stressful situation?"

She then told me about the mass the doctor had detected in her breast that was going to be biopsied the next day. "I know it's probably just a cyst, but I would appreciate your prayers," she shared with me. I could hear in her voice that she was smiling as she spoke.

Tanya's cycle is a familiar one:

- *An event occurs that could be frightening or upsetting.*
- *Resulting emotions arise from the painful event (in this case, anger, sadness, and fear).*
- *We resort to our habit of suppressing our emotions and pretending everything is alright.*
- *We eat off-program sweets in order to soothe ourselves.*

"It sounds like you're smiling right now, Dear One," I said. She acknowledged that she was.

"Are you smiling on the inside, too?" She admitted she was not.

We talked about what she was learning from High-Way 4 - that anger, sadness and fear were natural reactions to the news she had received.

We also talked about eating as the **symptom - not the cause** of her pain, and that she could look at her cravings as the tip of the iceberg, and her emotional pain as the part of the iceberg underneath the surface. Until the underlying issues were faced and felt, nothing could change.

Her cyst was benign, thank heavens, and she found a new coping skill - awareness and acceptance of her feelings - to replace her old guilt and shame when cravings arose.

I'm so grateful for the Tanyas in this program - women and men who are working the High-Ways every day to learn to love and accept themselves and their emotions more fully.

Our Fear of Feelings

As a society we allow our young children to feel without shame. When we hear the sadness or anger in a hungry baby's cry, they are seen as normal and natural, and we are led to respond with love. Yet most of us receive a message as we grow older that one or both of these emotions are no longer "acceptable."

By the time we reach adulthood, "shoulds" about our emotions have taken hold. Look carefully at this quote from a health magazine and guess why it concerns me:

> *"People who compulsively overeat are those who use food as their way of coping with negative emotions."*
>
> – Joseph Goldberg, MD

Did you catch it? He called some emotions negative. I beg to differ.

Releasing "Bad" Feelings Forever

Most of us grew up being taught to label certain feelings as bad, especially Mad and Sad. Recognize these phrases?

"Your father's in a bad mood."
"I feel bad about what happened."
"You shouldn't be angry about that little thing."
"Don't cry. You'll upset the others."
"Don't raise your voice to me."
"Stop crying or I'll give you something to cry about."

Most of us have been programmed to judge our feelings as "bad." Is it possible to turn around our thinking and see anger and sadness as the gifts that they are? It is. Information leads to transformation.

Dr. Martin Luther King started his worldwide social justice movement on his angriest day. Yet we would not call him mean.

Dr. King wept almost every night of his adult life for the 21 friends he buried before he himself was buried. Would we call him weak? Just the opposite.

Heroes like Dr. King have much to teach us.

The Fire and Water of Feelings

I find it helps to think of Mad and Sad as two elements in nature: **fire and water.**

When we are angry we use phrases like "hot under the collar" or "boiling mad" or say that the team is getting "fired up" before the game. In *8 to Your IdealWeight* we combine anger and energy and call this fiery passion **Angergy,** our energy for change.

Anger = Fire

"Angergy"

While fire energy is healthy and natural, it must be balanced. When there is too much fire, we need water. **Sadness is our water energy.** Think of it as your **Release,** and use it to let go and say goodbye. What you may not realize, is that through the water of your tears, you are releasing toxins and stress.

Sadness = Water

"Release"

The thing we have misunderstood about Mads and Sads is that we always have them at the same time and to the same extent. We have never had one without having an equal amount of the other. Yet most of us are unaware of the one we are suppressing. We hide it, even from ourselves, because we are less comfortable with it.

When we repress feeling our sadness (water energy), our fire takes over and turns to rage. When we stuff and suppress our feelings of anger (fire), we lose our passion, and our sadness (water) takes over. Too much sadness/release leads to depression.

How much energy do we have when we're depressed? None, because we have cut ourselves off from our **angergy**. How much peace do we have when we're raging? None, because we have cut ourselves off from our **sadness**.

The good news is simple, **we can learn to feel all our feelings again.**

Anita's Story

Anita came to me for coaching at the request of her mother who was concerned about her daughter's depression. I listened as Anita told me about her sorority sister taking her own life just a few months before. She shared that now that she was home for the summer, her mother was on her constantly about sleeping too much, having a messy room, etc.

What Anita's Mom didn't realize was the natural cycle of grief. We need time and space to feel our strongest feelings, but it can alarm those around us who want us to behave in a more "normal" way. Remember, sadness is not energy, it is release of energy. Feeling a need for more sleep is absolutely natural and healthy during the grieving process.

At the same time, it's important to feel not only our sadness about our losses, but our natural angers about them. I suggested to Anita that she write three letters expressing her anger and sadness: one to her former sorority sister, one to her mom, and one to herself, and then burn them. As she touched her emotional truth she would feel whole again and make her best decisions moving forward.

She and her Mom were very grateful for how much better she "felt" after she did.

Normal is nothing but the setting on a dryer.

Releasing Our "Shoulds" About Feelings

As this program unfolds, many Ideals realize that they want to set a boundary with someone - their spouse, their parents, their boss, or even their adult children. Yet, they have an underlying belief that they "shouldn't" be angry at loved ones or set limits with friends because of "all they have done for me."

What if we didn't get mad at a neighbor who was harming our pet because we didn't want to upset them? It's hard to imagine anything so ludicrous. Yet we hold back when it comes to standing up for ourselves like we stand up for those in our care. The good news is that we can start honoring our feelings, setting boundaries, and taking care of ourselves beginning now.

I've also had Ideals tell me they felt guilty feeling sad or mad because "others have it worse off." This is a misunderstanding of how our hearts work. We can't talk ourselves into feeling or not feeling. We either do or do not feel sad or angry, and when we do, the healthiest gift we can give ourselves is to allow and embrace it.

To Feel is to Heal.

Have you seen Pixar's animated film **Inside Out**? The writers worked with the top researchers in the world of emotions to put together the script. One of those researchers, Paul Ekman, shared this with the *New York Times:*

"Studies find that it is anger (more so than a sense of political identity) that moves social collectives to remedy injustice... Meanwhile, we might be inclined to think of sadness as a state of inaction and passivity — the absence of any purposeful action. But **Inside Out** offers a new approach to sadness: Embrace sadness. Let it unfold. **It will move you.**"

Is it Feeling or "BCing"?

Ideals often ask:

"You say when we're blaming and complaining we're giving our power away, and yet you say to feel all our feelings. How do we do both?

It's a good question. When you are expressing your feelings repeatedly, in the break room or in front of a television set, and taking no action to remedy the situation, you are BCing, Blaming and Complaining.

When you express your feelings once or twice to get clear about how you feel, and then take action (Acting and Dreaming), then you are allowing your feelings to "move you" in a healthy way. Unlike BCing, ADing will take you up the Power Pyramid.

How We Run From Our Feelings

Judgment never feels good, and the last thing we want to judge is our emotions. When we judge our feelings as bad, we look for a way to "run from" them with food, alcohol, cigarettes, overwork, etc. We can even use exercising excessively to run from our feelings.

But when we're running from our feelings it's a no-win situation because painful feelings can only be outrun for so long. One day we'll explode into rage, implode into depression, or find ourselves battling pain and sickness. Some physical ailments that have been associated with suppressed anger include fevers, (burning up), rashes, headaches, back aches, TMJ, anxiety attacks, urinary infections, acne, spasms and high blood pressure.

In order to feel good, we have to feel.

To stay healthy, we can learn to recognize how we "Run from" our feelings. Here's a list of some of the ways **we suppress our emotions:**

> Blame - "You make me angry..."
> Analyze - "Why?"
> Apologize - "I'm sorry I'm crying"
> Deny - "I'm too tired to be angry about it"
> Defend - "I have a right to be angry!" (Yes you do.)
> Fix - "I have to go shopping so I'll feel better again"
> Obsess - Telling five people in one day how angry you are at her/him
> Run - Hiding. Not checking in with your partner, not weighing weekly, etc.
> Use - Using food to stuff your feelings deeper and deeper within.

Yes, they spell B-A-A-D-D-F-O-R-U. Which of the above do you recognize in yourself?

> *"The first step toward change is awareness.*
> *The second step is acceptance."*
>
> - Nathaniel Branden,
> author of *"Six Pillars of Self-Esteem"*

How to Feel Better

"What has occurred throughout the course of your day is much less significant than how you feel about it. Anything that has occurred in your past is not nearly as important as how you feel about it now. By telling the truth about how you feel in any moment, you are putting yourself in touch with what is most significant in that moment. You have to tune in to how you feel in order to express it honestly and clearly. Only after you tune in can you allow yourself the freedom to choose to feel something else."

- Daniel Scranton

When you are ready to release the dam of "shoulds" and start to feel all your feelings again, here are 8 Avenues to accepting your emotions and opening your heart:

1. Walk it through.

2. Talk it through.

3. Write it through.

4. Movie Night it through.

5. Art it through.

6. Heart it through.

7. Pray it through.

8. Meditate it through.

1. Walk it through.

Sometimes when I'm angry, I find myself heading for the door for a walk (always alerting those I'm with that I'll be back.) On my most stressful days, I head to the tennis courts to slam a ball at a wall. It is a powerful energy release.

2. Talk it through.

Whether it's with a coach, a counselor, or a trusted friend or sibling, having someone who will listen without judgment or advice is an invaluable asset for the healing of the human heart.

3. Write it through.

A safe and powerful way to honor your feelings is by expressing them on paper. Be aware that hanging onto that paper after you're finished may cause a challenge if others read it. That's why I suggest we be raw in our honesty on paper, with no edits or withholds, and then burn it.

4. Movie night it through.

In the Resource section at the end of this book, there is a list of emotion-releasing films that have helped me process and feel my feelings. Whether it's on your computer or going to a movie theatre by yourself, movies can be very moving.

"Couldn't keep it in, heaven knows I tried..."

– from the Disney movie *"Frozen"*

5. Art it through.

As a composer of over 100 songs, I have written my best music at my highest and lowest points. My artist friends say the same. Let your emotions flow through you and release any concerns about the perfection of the final outcome. Just feel and express.

6. Heart it through.

Sometimes sitting and letting your emotions flood into your heart is the most healing and loving act we can take.

Feelings are suppressed by busy-ness. They are released when we allow ourselves the gifts of stillness and silence.

7. Pray it through.

If you believe, as I do, that there is someone who is always listening - Jesus, an angel, or a loved one who has passed - talking to them in prayer can bring powerful peace.

8. Meditate it through.

Meditation is the release of thoughts and attachment. Sitting and focusing on your breath for five or ten minutes can calm your spirit and make room for your heart to heal. Or you may choose a simple phrase to repeat silently with each breath such as, "I honor and acknowledge my feelings as sacred."

For more on how to move up the Power Pyramid of feeling good, go to www.8toyouridealweight.com/recipes4life.

10 Ways to Find Comfort When You're Feeling Sad

I loved hearing from Karen about how she stood up for her feelings.

"When the big day came for my daughter's wedding, I started crying while they were taking her picture. One of my granddaughters said, 'Oh Grammy, don't cry.' I was so proud that I stood up for myself and said, 'I'm feeling all my feelings,' and I let the holy water flow. She chuckled with me and now knows it's okay to feel."

When you're wanting to honor your sadness here are some options:

1. Roll up in a fuzzy blanket and take a nap.

2. Take a bubble bath (scented candles optional).

3. Get a massage.

4. Have a Girls' Night Out where you paint pictures (there are businesses where you can do this in most major cities).

5. Ask for/give someone a hug.

6. Prepare a small bag of pistachios and watch a three-Kleenex movie like "*Notebook*" or "*A League of Their Own*" or one of my favorites, "*E.T.*"

7. Go for a walk in nature.

8. Listen to songs that help you touch your heart like "Mad World" by Michael Andrews, or Bonnie Raitt's "I Can't Make You Love Me," or practically any song by Adele.

9. Color in a coloring book. There are hundreds of adult coloring books out now.

10. Find a good counselor, minister or coach to talk to.

As you start to feel a bit better, take a deep breath and watch this Gratitude video:

"A Good Day" with Brother David Steindl-Rast

http://tinyurl.com/jbbc7dz

10 Healthy Ways to Express Your Anger

I was so grateful that Beth felt comfortable sharing her anger with me in an email:

"I don't think I smiled at all yesterday. I know I should be jumping for joy because what they found isn't cancerous. I am grateful for that, but I am so upset to be having another surgery. Splitting me wide open...again. Surgery number six. And I have to find a time that doesn't interfere with the plans I've already made. Every time I feel so homebound. I can't drive for a week. I can't do anything because I'll be hurting. I've just been through this so many times. This stupid growth is ruining my summer. I had plans to really do extra things with the kids and some just for me. Sorry I'm on a soap box."

I told her there was no need for an apology and encouraged her to really let herself feel her disappointment about her disrupted summer plans. It was so healthy and healing.

Here are 10 Avenues for releasing your Angergy:

1. Throw ice cubes at sidewalks.

2. Punch a pillow while yelling "It's not okay!"

3. Watch a movie about someone who was angry and used it to change their life. (See the Resource section at the end of the book.)

4. Go for a walk or a run.

5. Listen to angergizing music, such as "Fight Song" by Rachel Platten, "Hero" by Mariah Carey, "Brave" by Sara Bareilles or "Roar" by Katy Perry.

6. Write a really angry note and then burn it.

7. If you believe it will help, after you write your first raw angry letter (#6), write an angry note to the person involved using "I feel" rather than "you" statements. Then read it to a friend you trust before sharing it. Only share it with who you're angry with in person or over the phone. Never email or text an angry letter. Put on your big girl panties and face your fears.

8. Create Art - a painting, a poem, a song, or chalk art on the sidewalk.

9. Volunteer somewhere or visit an elderly neighbor. Listening to someone else's pain can help you unhook from your own.

10. Clean. This can be amazingly therapeutic. Find a pile of papers or magazines and release whatever no longer serves you.

Feeling With vs. Feeling For

Empathy is not doing the feeling work for someone. It's feeling with them.

Feeling for someone:

Over the years, I've had many conversations with parents who are upset with their teen's decisions. The challenge was that the parents were often more angry than the child, which had the opposite effect from what was intended. When the parents carried all the anger, the son or daughter did not connect with his/her own angergy and did not have the necessary energy to change.

For women in domestic violence situations, I often ask the parents or siblings to only share good qualities about the abuser for 30 days. This allows the abused daughter/sister to be angry enough herself that she will change her situation.

The same goes for spouses who get angry "for" their partner about an injustice being done to them. Carrying another person's anger for them guarantees that the imbalance continues and necessary growth is delayed.

When we overdo, you can be sure others will underdo.

Feeling with someone:

When we're training our coaches for this program, we review setting emotional boundaries. If one of my coaches is losing sleep worrying about an Ideal, I know she's draining her own resources unnecessarily. Compassion is healthy, worry is not.

We also coach them in phrases to avoid, such as "I understand." Each person is unique, and although we might have had a similar experience, such as the death of a loved one or a pet, each person's response is entirely unique to that relationship.

 Heartwork for High-Way 4

1. Create an "emotion timeline" for your life in your journal.

    A. While you were growing up, how were your emotions treated? Write about specific instances.

    B. At this point in your life, where are you in acceptance of your own emotions and the emotions of others?

C. If you were to be more open-hearted and honoring of your mads or sads, what might that look like?

2. If there is a feeling you have been suppressing lately, write a letter and apologize. It might sound like this:

"Dear feeling of _____ (name it)

I know I have not been giving you enough time lately. You are a gift to me because _____ I will do my best not to run away from you again."

Let it know, like you would a small child, that you can see the gift it has to give you.

We can replace thoughts of, "I shouldn't be feeling this way" with, "It's healthy and natural for me to feel this way."

 Partner/Reflection Questions

For your sharing this week, consider discussing the following:

1. The emotion I've had the hardest time accepting lately is...

2. Read any letters or excerpts of letters from your journaling or Heartwork that you feel comfortable sharing.

"The best and most beautiful things in the world cannot be seen or even touched. They must be felt with the heart."

- Helen Keller

HIGH-WAY 5:
HONEST COMMUNICATION

"Say what you need to say..."

- John Mayer,
musician

I'm so grateful for those who encouraged me to find my voice, which started with speaking up, saying no, and asking for what I wanted. Now I want to encourage you to do the same: to find the healthiest way to express yourself while taking full responsibility for your feelings.

In this chapter, we're going to speak in "I" instead of "you" language, as we learn:

- *How to ask for what we want in a clear and non-threatening way*
- *How to handle unsolicited advice*
- *How to turn off triangulation (3rd party communication)*
- *How to avoid defensiveness in arguments*
- *How to handle comments from family and friends*

The 4 Principles of Honest Communication

First, let's set a foundation with these overarching tenets:

1) By trying never to hurt anyone, we often end up hurting ourselves and other people.

2) Not letting others know how we feel and what we think is a form of dishonesty. When we do not tell others how their behavior negatively affects us, we are denying them the opportunity to change their behavior.

3) Because no one can know the thoughts or feelings of another, in taking Full Responsibility, the only person we can speak for is ourselves.

4) Everyone has the right to ask for what they want, refuse requests, feel and express anger, fear and hurt, make mistakes in order to learn, have opinions that are different from those of their family and friends, be treated as capable adults, and have their needs be as important as anyone else's.

Let's get started...

How to Ask For What We Want

This basic life skill is chronically weak in many adults. When we don't know how to ask, we end up resorting to phrases such as, "How come you never...?" or "Why do you always...?" which do nothing but put the receiver on the defensive.

By following a few clear cut guidelines, you'll be amazed how much more receptive others are to your requests. As one CEO told me, *"MK, if you could get my staff to start asking for what they want using these skills, it would be worth a million dollars to my business."*

So let's start with a simple tried and true formula for asking for what you want.

"When _____ I felt _____because _____.
Therefore, _____."

Simple, right? But there are four common errors that can derail the outcome by putting the other person on the defensive.

1. "When _____" The common mistake with this step is to lump events together. Listing multiple grievances implies that they always do this behavior. Stick to one example of the upsetting incidence, or if you must show a pattern, never mention more than two. More than two can feel overwhelming to the receiver's brain and flood them with emotions.

2. "I felt _____" Here it's important to share actual feeling words. It's easy to avoid sharing our feelings by replacing them with thoughts and opinions. If the word "that" follows "felt/feel" it is really a thought and not a feeling, such as "I felt that you didn't care about ..." That's not our feeling, it's our opinion.

3. "Because _____" This might sound like, "Because it seems like my opinion isn't really valued." To avoid making judgements like "Because you never listen to me" (ouch!) add the phrase "it seems" or "it looks like."

4. "Therefore _____ " This final phrase is optional. It can be a request for a change, a request for a further discussion, or something as simple as "I just wanted you to know. Thanks for listening."

When you put all these steps together, they are a thousand times more likely to be heard and responded to in a positive way:

"When we schedule date nights a few days in advance I feel loved and valued because I really look forward to our one-on-one time."

This form of asking for what we want is much riskier than blaming someone else or stuffing our feelings, so remind yourself of High-Way 2: *No Risk, No Reward.*

How to Handle Unsolicited Advice

When I was 35, my father gave each of us kids $5,000. "I want to watch my inheritance bless your lives, not wait until after I'm gone," my wise Dad told us.

It was 1988 and I decided to purchase a used Honda Civic I had found for that price. Two days after I told him my intentions, I got a long letter about how buying American was so much better for the economy and that I should consider changing my mind.

I called him, thanked him for the letter, and shared my feelings.

"Dad, thanks for your letter. I can tell you put a lot of thought into it. I can also tell you feel really strongly about it. I feel just as strongly about purchasing a car that gets good gas mileage. None of the American made used cars can touch Honda in that regard. So, if this money came with strings attached, and I need to use it for something you approve of, I understand, and can send you back the money. Just let me know."

He was quiet for a minute, and then said, "Go ahead and buy your Honda, honey. It's your money to use as you want."

I thanked him for his generosity.

When others tell us what we should do, my two favorite responses are, "Thank you. I will take that into consideration," and "I acknowledge your position and promise to weigh it carefully before I make my decision."

I recall a priest friend of mine who left the priesthood at the age of 44. During his final sermon, these words stuck with all of us:

"Concerning my decision, I have discovered that for those who do not know me, no explanation is enough, and for those who truly know me, no explanation is necessary."

How to Turn Off Triangulation (3rd Party Communication)

This next skill made a huge difference in my life. We've all experienced it. Someone (X) tells a friend (Y) something that upsets them about someone else (Z). It's called "3rd Party Communication" but it is no party.

I believe that this X-Y-Z does more harm than almost any other communication habit around. The great news is that **you** can stop it in its tracks by determining which role you are playing: X, Y or Z, and changing how you communicate. When you change your part in the trio, the strangulation of triangulation is ended.

Let's use an example:
X, Y, and Z at Work

Co-workers AleXis (X) and Yolanda (Y) were comfortable in their jobs. After all, they'd been working there for over twenty years. What they did not like was change. So when a younger woman, Zandra (Z) was hired as their peer and brought a lot of new ideas, they felt threatened.

AleXis was most bothered by how Zandra would quote research when she brought up new ideas. She thought it was showing off and didn't like feeling talked down to. She would regularly complain to Yolanda about the new office "know-it-all."

One day as they were waiting for a meeting to start, Yolanda found herself alone with Zandra, and decided to give her new co-worker a little advice. She shared with her that AleXis was tired of all her quoting research to show how smart she was and that unless she wanted to upset her more, she'd best stop suggesting so many improvements.

Zandra was shocked and deeply hurt. If AleXis had hidden resentments toward her, maybe everyone did! From that day on Zandra tried to bite her tongue at meetings, but found her trust was so damaged that she eventually asked for a transfer.

Can you see what each individual could have done to prevent the outcome?

The Solution

As the saying goes, it takes two to tango. I like to add that it takes three to *tangle*. The great news is that it only takes one to *de-tangle*! No matter who you are in this triangle of trouble, you can stop X-Y-Z all by yourself for good. Here's how:

If you are X (AleXis), go directly to Z (Zandra). "Z, have you got a minute? There's something I'd like to talk about." You can then follow it with something like, "When this happens _____, I feel a little uncomfortable, because it seems _____."

If you're Y (Yolanda), when X comes with her complaint, simply tell her to go talk to Z. Even if X says, "Oh no, Z would never listen," just be a broken record. "You need to talk to Z. There's nothing I can do about it. You need to talk to Z." She'll eventually get the hint and stop BCing.

Finally, if you're Z (Zandra), a great de-tangler phrase is simply asking the messenger, "So, Y, do you agree?" Person Y never carries a message she doesn't agree with on some level, so she is using X as an X-cuse to tell you what she (Y) thinks. Rather than being your best friend in this situation, Y is almost always *your biggest problem.*

In my experience with this, which has diminished greatly now that I have this skill, middle person Y will sometimes even make up statements that X said that are far from the truth. When I'm Z, on a few occasions I've gone to X to try and "clear things up." X usually looks at me quizzically and says, "What are you talking about?"

There you have it. It's all within your power. Happy de-tangling!

How to Avoid Defensiveness in Arguments

The main cause of anger is easy to guess...feeling disrespected. So, it begs the question, what is the most respectful thing we can do for another person?

The answer is: listen.

It's a worn out phrase between clashing personalities: "You're not listening to me." While we hear it from teenagers to their parents, or customers to customer service agents, perhaps the most destructive instance is when difficulties in listening are a problem between spouses.

One of the greatest causes of divorce is "the inability to resolve conflicts." If one or both partners aren't feeling respected and heard, ground rules and guidelines can help restore harmony.

Years ago, an Imago therapist taught me a simply powerful listening skill, which I adapted using the letters: L.A.D.I.I.

Using L.A.D.I.I. for Open-Hearted Listening

The next time you receive a *compliment or a critique*, try using this simple formula to be sure you're hearing what they're saying. . (Note: Always make sure the other person has time to give you their full attention.)

L. Let me see if I got this...

A. Acknowledge what they said, using as many of their words and phrases as possible.

D. Did I get that?

(Wait for their reply)

I. Is there more?

(Wait for their reply)

I. I can Imagine that feels...

Using L.A.D.I.I. to Accept Compliments

It's good to start off practicing using the L.A.D.I.I. technique to accept compliments.

It's amazing how many times in an average week we'll receive a compliment, and then brush away the affirming words with, "I'm only doing my job," or "This old thing?" We are like the plant on a windowsill with the shades drawn. There is sunlight outside but we're not letting it in.

At the same time, pushing away compliments discourages the sender from ever sending them again. Giving a verbal compliment can be risky, and the sender may end up feeling foolish for reaching out. Rather than discourage them, acknowledge the compliment using L.A.D. "Let me see if I got that. You're really grateful I got up early to make you breakfast. Did I get that?"

Then once you've practiced using L.A.D. a few times to accept a compliment, practice all five steps when hurt feelings arise. Below is an example of what that looked like for one Ideal:

L.A.D.I.I. for Working Through Challenges:

Wife: Honey, I'd like to use LADII to talk with you about the cookies you brought home from work today. Do you have five minutes?

Husband: Sure. (He may ask to see a sheet of paper with the 5 steps listed.)

Wife: When you brought home my favorite kind of cookies when you know I've just started the IdealWeight program, I felt confused and a little angry.

Husband: Let me see if I'm getting this. When I brought those cookies home, you felt angry and confused. Did I get that?

(Notice, the listener here must resist the temptation to defend himself with "facts.")

Wife: Yes. You know they're my favorites and that I'm on this program of reducing my sugars. I couldn't understand why you'd do something like that.

Husband: I know you're on this program and it doesn't make sense that I'd do something like this. Did I get that?

Wife: Right.

Husband: Is there more?

Wife: Not right now. Thanks for listening.

Husband: I can imagine that was confusing Sweetheart. I'm so sorry. Honestly, you've been so strong in your program that I didn't even think you'd be tempted. I forgot they're your favorites. If I would have brought them home with aluminum foil over the top, would that have helped?

Wife: That would have been much better. And from now on,

let's put any sweet treats in the cupboard so I don't have to see them when I walk by them. Most days I don't have cravings, but when I'm really tired...I just don't want them within sight, does that make sense?

Husband: Makes sense. I'll do that. You look great these days, by the way!

Wife: Let me see if I got that... (laughter) :)

Note: If the person is letting you know their feelings were hurt, after you use L.A.D.I.I., you can use **The A.A.A. Formula:** Admit, Apologize and Offer Amends - suggesting two or three possible solutions to see if any of them would help resolve the issue and/or soothe their feelings.

As formal as this skill may seem, my partner and I have loved using it. I've also shared it with hundreds of couples who agree - it helps to have a formula to follow for open-hearted listening.

"The first duty of love is to listen."

- Paul Tillich

How to Handle Comments from Family and Friends

Would you rather be right, or would you rather be happy?

Over the years, Ideals have asked for skills to handle challenging questions or comments from those closest to them. Sometimes these comments from loved ones can trigger us into feeling defensive. Just remember that no one wakes up intending to be hurtful that day. Then practice responding in a way that avoids an argument while retaining your power.

It's good to start with releasing the need to be right or change their minds. We can accept what they say as true for them in this moment. While we don't need to be "nice" and weaken our truth, we can be kind, even when they're not. Rather than getting defensive, we can assume they mean well.

Here are some responses that may be helpful:

1. "Have you lost weight?"

You can have some fun with them by saying, "I stopped losing weight because I don't want to find it again. Now I release my extra weight, and yes I have!"

2. "How much have you lost?"

"More and more" or "All that I wanted" seem to work well if you're not comfortable sharing your scale numbers.

3. "How have you done it?"

I have heard Ideals respond with, "Using a really simple Get Real health program. It's called '8 to Your IdealWeight.' If you'd like to take me out for coffee or lunch sometime I'd love to tell you all about it."

4. "Why are you on a diet? You don't need to lose weight."

"Thanks for the compliment! I'm not on a diet, I just eat healthier these days. I appreciate your support." (Then change the subject.)

5. "Is this one of those fad diets?"

"It's definitely not a diet because it feels so good I won't be going "off" it. (Then change the subject.)

6. "You can't eat this way forever!"

"I'm only doing it one day at a time. Wanna play a game of cards?"

7. "Are you saying sugar is bad?"

"I didn't say it was. In fact, I still have some in small quantities. I've noticed I have lots more energy these days. Speaking of energy, want to go for a walk?"

8. "I suppose you're going to tell me I need to go on it, too."

"I would never do that. **8 to Your IdealWeight** is only for people who really want it, and it doesn't seem like a priority for you right now. I love you just the way you are."

9. "You won't stick with it; you never do."

"I can see with my track record how you'd say that. Before I was on diets. This is a way of eating for life. Time will tell. Want to go for a walk?"

No matter what, do your best to see yourself wearing a crown and hold your head high...

Heartwork for High-Way 5

1. Use L.A.D.I.I to listen to someone this week. Journal about how the process felt and how the interaction went.

2. Ask for what you want from someone. It could be as small as asking for someone to put the wash in the dryer, or to go for a walk, or to practice L.A.D.I.I. with you.

 Partner/Reflection Questions

For your sharing this week, consider listening to your partner using L.A.D.I.I. as she shares her answers to any of the following:

1. The person I have the hardest time listening to without getting triggered is...

2. The person I have the most trouble speaking my truth to is:

3. The person I X-Y-Z with the most is:

4. One thing I could do/am doing to improve my communication is...

HIGH-WAY 6: FORGIVENESS OF THE PAST

*"The weak can never forgive.
Forgiveness is the attribute of the strong."*

- Gandhi

Two Stories, One Healing

As painful as the next two stories are, I hear stories like them all the time from Ideals. For so many of us, there came a day in our young lives when all other means of protection or emotional expression seemed out of reach, so we resorted to the one thing we had complete control over - how much we ate - to balance the power struggle.

Elaine can remember the day. She was 11 and her alcoholic and abusive father was walking with her and her brother down the main street of their small town. As an overweight woman passed them on the sidewalk he muttered, "I hate fat slobs." Eleven-year-old Elaine decided in that moment that she would gain weight to get her revenge against him.

Stephanie had no idea that her past was the trigger for her weight issues. What she did know was that her pre-diabetic diagnosis was scary, and she didn't want to model carrying 50 extra pounds for her two kids, so she came to one of my IdealWeight lectures. That day I spoke about how we unknowingly carry emotional weight from the past on our physical bodies.

After the talk, she waited until everyone else had left to ask me, "How do we find out if we're carrying around our past?" I invited her to sit down with a pad and pen and complete one phrase 10 times: "The good thing about hanging onto this extra weight is ..."

Without writing a word she said aloud, "I'd be promiscuous. When I was 19 I did things I wasn't proud of. I would never do that to my kids."

I invited her to go for a walk with me, during which she began to see how that 19-year-old had grown up and become a responsible 31-year-old. With a glimmer of hope that things could be different now, she signed up for the course, and over the next eight weeks did the work of unhooking her bright future from her darker past. Because she was willing to use the laser beam light of awareness to melt her iceberg beneath the surface, she eventually released 55 pounds of heaviness and a decade of shame.

Both Elaine and Stephanie felt imprisoned, not realizing that they alone held the key that would open the prison's door - forgiveness.

Why Forgive? My Father's Parting Gift

I watched my father forgive some important people in his life in his dying days. When I saw the peace it brought him, I decided I wasn't waiting. I wanted to forgive and find that freedom and peace.

These days I sleep like a baby, don't get colds, flus or headaches, and I've written and burnt over 25 forgiveness letters over the past 30 years. Is it possible there is a connection?

According to a 2014 Johns Hopkins Research study, the act of forgiveness reaps huge rewards for your health, lowering the risk of heart attack; improving cholesterol levels and sleep; and reducing pain, blood pressure, and levels of anxiety, depression and stress.

The Stanford University Forgiveness Project headed by Dr. Fred Luskin found even more benefits to forgiveness:

- *More energy*
- *Better decision making*
- *Better chance of achieving your dreams*
- *Fewer incidences of cancer*
- *Stronger immune systems*
- *Less muscle tension and related disorders such as TMJ*

My insights from personally coaching hundreds of Ideals also show that the act of forgiveness dramatically speeds up weight loss. Science agrees. When we hold a grudge we activate the stress response, which floods the body with the stress hormones cortisol, adrenaline, and insulin, ultimately making it easy and convenient for the body to store fat around the middle - 'belly fat.'

Clearly, the price of unforgiveness is high, costing us our health, happiness and serenity.

We have all had life challenges. Mine have included embezzlement by a trusted friend, losing a college roommate to sudden death, being in a violent marriage, having my 8th grade daughter stalked by a man with a gun, and discovering my former partner was having an affair. Through it all forgiveness hasn't always been easy for me, but it has been simple, and powerfully life-changing.

"The most self-loving thing you can do for yourself is to forgive other people."

- Dr. Dean Ornish,
author of *"Eat More, Weigh Less"*

Heart is Where the Home Is

Before I give you 3 simple steps to forgiveness and one simple formula, let me paint a picture...

Imagine you and your spouse just got married and the two of you bought a new home. At first you enjoy decorating it with things you love - things that bring you joy. But over time, the basement starts to fill up with junk. Broken items, worn out furniture, things the kids leave behind when they head to college, and the items you offered to store for a neighbor start to accumulate. Pretty soon all that clutter leaves no room for anything else, and even starts to smell. You know a really good cleaning would help, but you're just too busy.

Now imagine your heart is that new home. Since birth you've been filling it with those you love. Yet along the way some of those trusted people said or did things that hurt you, and with each unforgiven incident, the painful memories residing in your heart sting whenever they come to mind.

Imagine this "heart clutter" growing over time. Guilt and resentment from emotional events that you didn't resolve when they happened start to fester. You'd love to have a clean heart, but it seems you "don't have time" to cleanse.

You also find yourself justifying the mess with thoughts like, "It's other people's junk!" You continue to wait for them to clean it up by apologizing...but they never do. The result?

You feel stuck with a heart full of hurt that has no room for new love, new joy or new compassion.

Today is a day to lighten your load, to decide that you are ready to feel better. The great news is, we are never stuck. We can take charge of our own heart cleanse.

In a few pages, I'll invite you to write a forgiveness letter. You will have a choice. As long as you hold onto regrets or resentments of others, the energy you could be using for fun or creative outlets will be tied up holding them prisoner. But one day you'll look and see...the real prisoner all along was you.

If you're thinking that they don't "deserve" to be forgiven, my invitation to you is this... don't forgive them for their sake. Forgive them for yours. **Forgiveness Frees.**

Defining Forgiveness

Unforgiveness is like taking poison and hoping the other person dies.

Before we write our letters, let's look at some of the misunderstandings about forgiveness. It is a concept rarely discussed, and when it is, the discussions are often reserved for hospital waiting rooms or funerals. It's time to get to know what it is and just how it works.

Forgiveness is...

- *the release of regret, resentment, and the desire for revenge*
- *moving your focus from the past to the present*
- *something you do for yourself, not the other person*

- *taking your power back*
- *refusing to live in the past*
- *a skill that can be learned*
- *freedom from the burdens of the past*
- *refusing to give the offender power over the present*
- *a choice*

Forgiveness is Not...

- *condoning a behavior*
- *letting them "get away with it"*
- *forgetting what happened*
- *denying your painful feelings*
- *reuniting or reconciling with the offender*
- *needing to trust them again*
- *understanding why they did it*

"If we really want to love, we must learn how to forgive."

- Mother Teresa

3 Steps of Forgiveness

Forgiveness is a conscious choice - a powerful tool that the happiest and most successful people use so often it becomes a *daily habit*.

To help you get started, I have broken it into three simple (but not always easy) steps:

1. Face it.
2. Feel it.
3. Forgive it.

Face It

"I keep wanting a month off to do my forgiveness work with my abuser," an Ideal shared with me. But very few of us are given that time. We must **make** time to do our healing work. For you it might mean a day at a retreat center, or an evening sitting by a lake or a bonfire. Wherever and whenever you do it, it can't be rushed. Feeling our feelings is often physically draining. Give yourself the time and space for this transformational work.

In the Bible, there is a beautiful explanation of this process in Ephesians:

Everything is shown up by being exposed to the light. Whatever is exposed to the light itself becomes light.

When we bring our secrets, regrets, resentments, and tears into the light, they become light and we become lighter.

Feel It

Once we face what happened, Step 2 naturally occurs - we Feel it. You know you are facing your painful past when the uncomfortable feelings around it resurface.

"But MK, don't you say to choose thoughts that feel good?" I have been asked. In order to feel good, we have to feel. Run to, not from, the feelings of your past. You don't have to like what happened, but you do have to accept it in order to be happy.

It happened. Now what are you going to do?

Pain cannot kill you, but the results of running from it can develop into addictions that can destroy not only your body, but your mind and spirit as well.

What you resist will persist.
What you embrace you can erase.

Forgive it

This final step happens in your heart, and can be affirmed when accompanied by an action. The healing ritual that acts as a phoenix rebirth for your new life is writing a forgiveness letter. Then, as a sign of your freedom, you will burn it.

But first, we need one more piece of the Forgiveness puzzle...

The Forgiveness Formula

"Forgiveness is a gift you give yourself. It frees you from the past and allows you to live fully in the present. When you forgive yourself and others, you are free."

- Louise Hay,
author of *"You Can Heal Your Life"*

Many years ago, I was blessed to learn a Forgiveness Formula that became a good friend to me. It lifted the weight of my past off my shoulders whenever I invited it in...

The Forgiveness Formula:
We were all doing the best we could at the time with the information we had.

If you're feeling any resistance to this formula, think back to something you regret. It could have happened yesterday or 20 years ago. Then ask yourself: *If I would have known then what I know now, would I have done it the same way?* The answer is always "No."

You were a good person then, doing the best you could at the time with the information you had. So, what do we need to do? Get more information! Why are you going through this **8 to Your IdealWeight** process? To get more information!

Once you can see how to forgive yourself, you can apply the process to any other person. The truth is that if they would have known then what you know now, **they wouldn't have acted that way.** But they may *never* know what you know now. That being the case, it doesn't have to *bind you in bitterness* to the past. You can choose to use your power to forgive.

Releasing Judgment of Others

It's so easy to think, "They should have known." But we don't know until we know.

To use a simple IdealWeight example, think about the last time you watched someone who was carrying quite a bit of extra weight sipping on what they considered a health drink which you knew to be over 100 grams of sugar in one drink. (Many that are sold by "health" outlets do have this much added sugar.)

You could get angry and tell them the dangers and they still would not be able to hear you until their hearts were ready.

People who hurt themselves or us only know what they know. Those who abuse were abused. Those who bully were bullied. Those who lie were lied to. Like an addiction to sugar, these are hard patterns to break.

The wonderfully freeing news is that you and I can break the cycle. You can end the need for revenge all by yourself. Instead of waiting for someone to apologize or reach out to you, release them in your heart, and on paper. Get to the point that you could see them across a room and not recoil. Find your peace. They really were doing the best they could, as hard as that often is to believe.

"If I would have known better, I would have done better."

- Maya Angelou,
author of *"I Know Why the Caged Bird Sings"*

The Hardest Person to Forgive

Many Ideals discover as they look back at things they haven't forgiven, that even when someone else hurts us, we still have to forgive ourselves for not standing up to them. Certainly this isn't true for a child who was abused, but as we grow older, many of us can look back at how we allowed people to "walk on us" without standing up for ourselves.

The best thing to do in that situation is release the weight of unforgiveness.

"Just because you've made mistakes doesn't mean that your mistakes get to make you. Forgive yourself and move on."

- Robert Tew

Writing Your Feelings and Forgiveness Letter

When you are ready to be free,
you can write the wrongs of your past

We humans resonate with symbolic action. The placing of a ring on a finger, the breaking of a glass, the pouring of water over the new member of the church, all of these are symbols that are held in high regard and rarely taken lightly.

Perhaps that is why the writing and burning of a Feelings or Forgiveness letter is so powerful. Somehow writing out the words of what it is we are releasing, and watching it go up in smoke is incredibly freeing. Here was a letter from an Ideal who experienced the power of this symbolic act.

"Writing the forgiveness letter changed my life. It was like I flipped a switch. I wrote mine to my in-laws and immediately felt the freedom from the weight I was carrying with me all that time. I didn't realize how much I was holding every day until I released it!

Since then I have written other forgiveness letters as well, and still have plans to write one to myself. I am the hardest on myself. I know that one will take time and I want to give it the time it deserves. Thank you so much for sharing this powerful process!"

- Heather S.

Letters of Release

Normally I write a **Forgiveness Letter** as my release letter, but sometimes I'm not yet ready to forgive. In that case I write a **Feelings Letter**. I give myself permission to get really angry with as many harsh words as I can muster. I let the person know on paper that what happened wasn't right or fair or moral or often even legal.

I find it's really healthy and healing to acknowledge the anger or hurt that resulted from their actions. When finished, I burn it, and feel so much lighter as a result.

A Feelings Letter is a good first step, but when you're ready to be completely done with the pain of what happened, I invite you to write a Forgiveness Letter. As with the Feelings Letter, it will be burnt to signify that you have released this person or past event and are free to live more fully in the present.

The Forgiveness Letter Process

1. Begin by selecting one person that you haven't forgiven. They may be living or deceased. They may even be a group of people. It could be God. It could be yourself.

2. Your Forgiveness Letter could start off with something like, "Dear So and So, I don't know why you did what you did, and truly, I really don't care why. As of today I am releasing you and freeing myself to move on with my life..."

3. When you're finished, sign it, fold it, put it in an envelope

and seal it. Write a big "F" on the front of the sealed envelope to signify "I Faced it, Felt it, and Forgave it. Now it's going in the Fire and I am Free!"

4. Finally, burn it. Charcoal grills and fireplaces work well for this powerful ritual.

You would never want to send the letter to the recipient to stir up old pain. This exercise is for you. Simply be grateful for your new release.

"I was so moved by the burning of my Forgiveness Letter that I spread the ashes over my garden. For me it symbolized the energy returning to earth to foster new life."

- Dani P.

The Forgiveness Test

How will you know if you've truly forgiven them? If you feel compassion for their losses and celebrate their success, you have forgiven them. If you celebrate their losses, you have not.

Apologies and Amends

"When you realize you've made a mistake, apologize immediately. It's easier to eat crow while it's still warm. "

- Dan Heist

The Forgiveness Letters are the sign that we have forgiven another, but what if we are the ones wanting to be forgiven by another?

Asking Forgiveness:

Apologies are powerful communicators, and should not be overused. Check to see if you are apologizing daily, and if so, take a deep breath before each apology to see if another response is more appropriate. For example, instead of saying, "I'm sorry I'm late," you can say, "Thank you for your patience."

However, for those times we let ourselves or someone else down by not keeping a promise or by doing something we regret doing, a sincere apology is in order.

Here are the three steps:

AAA: Admit. Apologize. Amend.

1. The first step is to admit that the hurt happened. Whether it was intentional or not, denial of any kind is likely to close the heart of the person who's feeling hurt.

2. The second step is to apologize. This can be as simple as, "I'm truly sorry," to "I'm so sorry I let you down. Can you forgive me?"

3. The third step is to make amends. Phrases such as "What can I do to make this up to you?" or "What can I do to show you how sorry I am?" are helpful. If the individual tells you that no amends are necessary, you can believe them. Not everyone needs this step of making restitution, but those who do have a hard time releasing what happened until it is received.

When Others Don't Apologize

"I've cut off with my father. I sent him a letter over a year ago saying I forgave him, but he never responded, so I'm done with him," the Ideal shared with me.

Do you hear it? She was still captive to her pain, waiting for her father to apologize. If true forgiveness is releasing regret, resentment and the need for revenge, she wasn't there yet. She still wasn't free.

When we haven't completely released a painful situation or person who hurt us, we are tied to them by an invisible rope around our hearts. Their actions take on amplified meaning, because we're giving them power over our peace by how they respond to us. If they respond, we're happier. If they don't, we're angrier. They have the control.

You can decide to take your power back from every hurtful decision today. Right now. Yes, it was unfair that it happened, but how fair is it that you're holding yourself back from happiness and peace after all this time?

We can choose to forgive them for not asking for or accepting our forgiveness. In releasing them and accepting what is, we will restore our freedom.

"Bitterness is like cancer. It eats upon the host. But anger and forgiveness are like fire. They burn all clean."

\- Maya Angelou

Heartwork for High-Way 6

Writing your Forgiveness Letter and burning it is all the Heartwork needed for this High-Way.

If you want to open your heart even more, here are some excellent films about forgiveness. Watch one and journal about it this week:

- *The Hiding Place*
- *Good Will Hunting*
- *Ordinary People*
- *As Good As It Gets*
- *On Golden Pond*
- *Eat, Pray, Love*

 ## Partner/Reflection Questions

For your sharing this week, consider discussing the following:

1. How has my unforgiveness been impacting my life?

2. How do I see my life changing as I unconditionally forgive myself and others?

3. What was it like to write and burn my forgiveness letter?

For more on Forgiveness, check out MK's TEDx talk, "The Most Important Question." Go to www.8toyouridealweight. com/recipes4life.

HIGH-WAY 7:
GRATITUDE FOR THE PRESENT

Growing up I thought of gratitude as...superfluous. It was something I did on thank you notes after my birthday because my Mom made me. To use food terms, it was butter on the cooked carrots, and I wasn't even sure I wanted the carrots.

Now I realize that gratitude is the entree in the banquet of a happy life. It is an exquisite and essential staple for a happy and healthy lifestyle. To be my best me, I have released the sweetness of sugar, and embraced the sweetness of gratitude.

Gratitude's Great-Full Benefits Are Free

Nobel Prize winner Hans Selye was a pioneer in stress research in the 1950's. In one of his studies, he identified the most beneficial and the most damaging emotions a person can have. His research showed that a "desire for revenge" created the most stressful damage in our bodies and that forgiveness is the key to releasing it.

Furthermore, Selye reported that **the most beneficial emotion was genuine gratitude.** When we appreciate, we create biochemicals in our bodies that are beneficial to rebalancing our bodily functioning. In other words, feeling grateful helps us to heal. There is obviously great physical benefit from regularly acknowledging our blessings with "an attitude of gratitude."

In *The Research Project on Gratitude and Thanksgiving*, the University of Miami team found that regular gratitude journaling or sharing increased energy, enthusiasm, and generosity, as well as the desire to exercise and greater commitment to reaching goals, *while reducing depression*. Additional studies have found that spending those last moments before bed jotting down some gratitudes can help us sleep better and longer.

Gratitude After A Loss

"MK, I am in need of some words of encouragement. I am tempted by emotional eating. I had two friends die this weekend and I just want to hide the sadness with food. It is just so hard having this happen. One was very unexpected and the other passed after a bout with breast cancer. I need help walking through these feelings. I am at work and with an office mate so I can't call anyone and won't be home tonight. Any help you can give me would be great."

- Joanie M.

When a relationship ends, there is always pain, whether it is through death or a break-up. When those hardest times in our lives show up, you certainly could distract yourself from your pain through food. No one would blame you but yourself. And that's the worst blame of all.

Just because we are hurt by someone doesn't mean we have to suffer or make them suffer.

While bringing closure with a friend, a family member or a romantic relationship is one of the most painful experiences we can face, we must face and feel it. I have found that the following letters can help us gently close the door and move on.

1. A letter of anger.

2. A letter of sadness.

3. A letter forgiving yourself (This letter is a Full Responsibility letter, which can include forgiving yourself for not loving yourself or them better along the way.)

4. A letter of forgiveness to them perhaps for dying so abruptly or so young.

5. A letter of gratitude for the good times

I have used these letters myself to say Goodbye to my father and loved ones. Sometimes it takes me a week to write them. Other times I write them all in a day. Gift yourself the time for healing. By releasing you will be one step closer to returning to your natural state of joy.

"What can you do right now to begin to turn your life around? The very first thing is to start making a list of things to be grateful for."

- Joe Vitale

A Gratitude Story from 9/11

One of the most powerful gratitude stories I've heard was shared on the Oprah show one year after 9/11. The woman had been a rescue worker, and for two days at the Twin Towers had worked on the rescue and recovery team amidst the debris and white dust.

Finally, she was forced to go home. Exhausted, she walked into her apartment and headed not for the bedroom or the refrigerator, but for the drawer in her office where she kept her writing materials.

"If I would have died three days ago, I would have died miserable," she wrote. "Today I am filled with the most overwhelming gratitude for life. I am therefore committing to write 3 gratitudes each day so that I never forget the gifts gratitude brings."

So what is the price tag of all of these amazing benefits that we would pay thousands for if it came in a pill? One minute each day for the rest of your life. That's how long sharing three gratitudes takes. Once you enter this wonder-filled world, you'll meet an amazing group who already live there - the happiest and healthiest people you know. And you'll be so grateful now that you do, too.

"I have renamed my bills. Now I refer to them as I.B.A.R.s.: Invoices for Blessings Already Received."

- Randy Gage

What Are You Waiting For?

What are you waiting for to get grateful?

Shawn Achor, in his phenomenal 2011 TEDx Talk on "The Happy Secret to Better Work," shares his research on a common misunderstanding. Most of us believe that if we work harder and are more successful we'll be happier. Then we'll be grateful.

Wrong, says the Harvard graduate. The reality is that successful people are happy first. Success, whether at weight release, relationships, jobs or sports, follows on the heels of happiness. And what does he recommend for greater happiness? Three new gratitudes each day.

"It's not the reality that shapes us, but the lens through which we view the world that shapes our reality."

- Shawn Achor,
author of *"The Happiness Advantage"*

Grateful for Our Bodies

If I told you the movie you just finished shooting was going to be a big hit, but that your body wasn't pretty enough, so the director was putting your head on someone else's body for the DVD cover, how would you feel?

Actually, this happens all the time to actresses. (I've never heard of it happening with actors, but I'm sure it does.) Any guesses who the most famous example of it is?

Julia Roberts. The movie? **"Pretty Woman."**

Is it any wonder that professional models have been shown in study after study to have the lowest self-esteem about their bodies of any group of women?

If we're waiting for the scale to reach a certain number to appreciate and feel good in our bodies, we've got it backwards. Successful long-term weight release is like all success. It is the result of happiness, not the cause. And as we have seen, happiness is the result of gratitude.

More Gratitude ⟶ More Happiness ⟶ More Success

*"Success is not the key to happiness;
happiness is the key to success."*

- Albert Schweitzer,
winner of the *Nobel Peace Prize*

The Gratitude Ritual

"You've never met an ungrateful person who is happy, nor have you ever met a grateful person who is unhappy."

- Zig Ziglar

The three most grateful groups on the planet are those who've come close to a loss, those who've had a loss, and those who know a loss is coming - like my father after his diagnosis with cancer. Every sunset and bird song became precious to him in those final months. I watched the peace it brought him, and decided I didn't want to wait for a diagnosis to find what he had.

Since then, the Gratitude Ritual is something I do *every day*. To review:

1. Sharing 3 things I'm grateful for from the past 24 hours

2. No repeats

Here are some questions Ideals have had about this ritual:

Does it work to share them over the phone? This one is tricky. If you do, have a set time that you will call each other, and have the same person initiate every day. Then, if the call goes to voicemail, the partner can call and leave her voicemail response as well.

Also, this must be a call **only** for sharing gratitudes and no longer than two minutes. This is not a check-in call or a time to discuss what you share. If you allow those to happen, the calls will extend to 5,10 or 15 minutes and you will soon decide you "don't have time." Every call is limited to two minutes. Honor that limit.

If 3 are good, why not 10 a day? Trust your coach and stick to three. My research has found that more than three are not sustainable. The goal for this Get Real program is long-term success. Three is the perfect number for daily acknowledgment, writing and sharing.

What am I supposed to be grateful for again? Anything that, if it were gone tomorrow, you would miss. We take so many things for granted. It will soon be easy for you.

Why the phrase, "from the past 24 hours?" The first week, you'll be grateful for what I call "The Biggies" - your kids, your spouse, your job, your health, etc.. After that, you'll want to be watching for "The Little Things."

This week I read gratitudes from others that included, "The feeling of my husband's hand on the small of my back," "My youngest granddaughter's giggles," and "My mom's great health at 89."

"Enjoy the little things, for one day you may look back and realize they were the big things."

- Robert Brault

No repeats? This is key. You don't want to get into a gratitude rut or it will stop feeling good after the 3rd or 4th time. Instead, look at life through a child's eyes and see it fresh every day. I've read some distinctly delightful gratitudes over the years, including:

- *That I now have a job where someone tells me to stop at the end of the day*
- *The inventor of the fly swatter*
- *Driving with the windows open*
- *My ability to whistle*
- *Coaches who care more about kids than scoreboards*

- *Pockets*
- *A hug just when I needed it*
- *That my parents gave me piano lessons*
- *The work of Heifer International to end world hunger in a sustainable way*
- *YouTube.com flashmob videos when I'm falling asleep at work (Heathrow Airport is one of my faves)*
- *The beauty and grace of Princess Kate*

Who should I share them with? I used to invite my kids to share them on the way to school with, "Do you want to go first or do you want me to?" Or you may want to invite gratitudes around the dinner table before diving into your meal. Either way, sharing doubles the fun as long as you remember not to "should" on anyone to join in.

My friend **Abby Goodlaxson** is a health teacher at a Midwestern high school. Since learning this skill at my training six years ago, she now emails her 3 daily gratitudes to the *dozen* Gratitude Groups she's started over the years: students, basketball teams, parents, fellow *8 to Great* trainers, etc.

None of us were surprised when she won the **2016 P.E. Teacher of the Year** for the State of Iowa and then went on to win the Regional award, making her one of 6 in the nation. She's one of the most vibrant and loving people I know, and I'm so grateful she is now a Master Trainer of these High-Ways.

You can, like Abby, find a small Gratitude Group, or share with that one special partner:

- *Your child at bedtime*
- *Your spouse before you get out of bed*
- *Your co-worker in Post-it notes*

- *Your sibling through emails*
- *Your teen in texts*
- *The world through social media*

I suggest social media as a bonus but not your mainstay for daily gratitude sharings because some days your gratitudes will be extremely personal. I have seen all of the following:

- *I'm grateful the CAT scan was clear*
- *I'm grateful I found a good divorce lawyer*
- *I'm grateful we had our pet for 15 wonderful years*

You can do gratitudes five days a week or every day. And remember, when you partner with just one person, they do not have to do the gratitudes with you. You can simply invite them to receive yours. You may want to warn them, however, they are contagious.

"Your life will change to the degree that you feel grateful. If you are a little bit grateful, your life will change a little bit. If you are very grateful, your whole life will change. If you live gratitude every single day, the light of your life will uplift the world."

- Rhonda Byrne,
author of *"The Secret"*

Mad-itudes and Grit-itudes

When sharing gratitudes, be on the watch for any "imposters."

True gratitudes are always for things that are, rather than things that "aren't." For example, you want to steer clear of sarcasm or put-downs. I call them **"Mad-itudes"** and they sound like: 'I'm grateful I finally got a compliment from my husband." "I'm grateful this stupid election is almost over." "I'm grateful my kids don't act like the neighbor's kids!"

The above examples are actually complaints in Gratitude disguise. They don't feel good to share or to hear. See them for what they are and gently turn your attention to those gratitudes that feel good.

"Grit-itudes" are, on the other hand, often very helpful. They are those appreciations we say when our frustrations are high or our energy is low. I sometimes will write 20, 30 or 50 on really hard days in order to turn my attitude back toward joy. They start off with the very basics:

I am grateful I can write.

I am grateful I can spell.

I am grateful that I can see.

I am grateful I am breathing.

I am grateful I have thought of 5 gratitudes so far and only have 45 to go.

You get the idea.

Of all the High-Ways, I hear Ideals say they are most grateful for two: Forgiveness and Gratitude. Sheri found a delightful adaptation as a single Mom:

"I loved learning the Gratitude Ritual and I found a fun way to use it at home. When my middle school boys start fighting, now I yell 'Gimme three!' and they have to both give me 3 things they're grateful for. It stops the fight every time! The miracle is that now they not only do the 3 gratitudes every day with me, but whenever they are fighting one of them will often turn to the other and shout out, 'Gimme three!' Such a blessing!"

- Sheri W.

The Gratitude Guarantee:
When you're grateful, you feel good.
When you feel good, good things happen.

Staying Grateful on the Journey to Your IdealWeight

"The reason most people give up is that they look at how far they still have to go instead of how far they have come."

- Terry League

I love being grateful for my little successes. As a small business owner, there are no gold watches in my future, so I celebrate and am grateful for the little wins along the way.

I encourage you to do the same.

One of the ways we celebrate in our IdealWeight Small Groups is by inviting Ideals to list 10 changes they are grateful for every time they reach a 10-pound goal.

Here is a list from an Ideal who is the mother of 4:

1. I am grateful I'm so unbelievably proud of myself! I smiled the whole time I was in the shower this morning after I weighed!

2. My clothes fit so much better and are soon going to look sloppy.

3. I'm grateful for how amazingly easy it's been.

4. I'm grateful that this program really is about willing power not willpower.

5. I can really see myself reaching my IdealWeight!

6. The *8 to Great* processes are such a help with the stresses of family life.

7. I'm grateful I'm staying calm even when all 4 of my kids act up at once!

8. I feel more rested in the mornings, ready to take on the day. Even getting to work a few minutes earlier than normal for me.

9. I'm grateful I'm more confident, walking a little taller. Even though I'm only 5'2"!

10. I'm grateful for my confidence and excited to share the good news with others!

Are you celebrating that you made it all the way to this chapter in the book? That you haven't thrown out this food program like you have so many others? Have a celebration! My favorite "Self-Giftings" include:

- *Getting a manicure, pedicure or facial*
- *Getting a massage*
- *A "Girls Weekend" at a hotel or resort*
- *Buying some sexy underwear or a fun new dress.*
- *Swinging on the swings or hitting balls in a batting cage.*
- *Going to my fave coffee shop with a fave romance novel*
- *Getting tickets to a concert or watching my favorite team play baseball (Go Royals!)*
- *Sleeping in and enjoying a healthy breakfast in bed.*
- *Getting a hot new hairdo.*
- *Hiring an organizer and telling her she gets $1 extra for every box of stuff that goes out the door with her.*

"I have released my first 20 pounds on 8 to Your IdealWeight. Meanwhile, this program has changed the way I think and the grateful way I look at life. My first dream has come true. I'm so grateful I have a lap for my new little granddaughter to sit on. Thank you to my small group Coach Peggy!"

- Julie G.

Gratitude for Couples

Many Ideals have asked me how to bring the Gratitude Ritual into their marriage. If your spouse is not open to sharing three gratitudes a day with you, be grateful for their honesty. Here are two other options to turn gravity into gratitude...

1. Write down one thing you appreciate about your partner on a notecard and leave it on his/her car dashboard or in their coat pocket a couple of times a week. Don't expect a notecard in return, simply give to them in order to soften your own heart and keep your perspective positive. If asked why you're doing it, one simple explanation is, "because it feels good to appreciate you."

2. If your spouse tends to be overly critical, it is often his/her *own* insecurity directed at you. Reinforce your own positive attitude by affirming him/her instead of falling into the criticism mode yourself. Acknowledge that you heard the statement with a phrase like, "I hear you asking for more home cooking. Thanks for letting me know. I get the sense this is pretty important to you." What they share next will be the real heart reason behind their statement.

When You Forget, Just FGH

Sometimes Ideals tell me they're reluctant to start the Gratitude Ritual because they have had a history of starting things they didn't finish. I like to remind them that this exercise soon feels so good you won't want to stop, but if you do forget for a day, a week, a month or a year, just FGH yourself:

- *Forgive yourself for forgetting*
- *Be Grateful you remembered*
- *Have Hope that you'll remember better next time.*

And begin again.

"What's important is that you enjoy and appreciate every day, and that's something you can accomplish by just living in the moment. Don't look behind you. Unless someone yells, "Look out behind you!" Then you should look. Otherwise, don't waste time looking behind or worrying about the future. Stay in the present.
There are a few ways to do that:

- *Stop and smell the roses.*
- *Wake up and smell the coffee.*
- *Enjoy the sweet smell of success.*

  (I guess it's a lot about your nose.)"

- Ellen DeGeneres

 Heartwork for High-Way 7

1. Share these 3 questions with at least 3 people this week:

They could be family, friends or co-workers. Simply let them know you're taking a course, and that it's your homework to ask and share the answers to these 3 questions with 3 people.

1. What is something I don't know about you?

2. What is something we agree on?

3. What is something you appreciate about me?

2. Take a risk and invite someone to be your gratitude partner after these 8 weeks are complete.

 Partner/Reflection Questions

For your sharing this week, consider discussing the following:

1. Discover the fun of creating an Avalanche of Appreciation about someone or some aspect of your life. Write at least 25 things you appreciate about that one thing or person. It could be focused on your child, your Mom or Dad, your grandchild, your home, your community, your job, your hobby, your hubby, etc.

Share some or all of the list with your partner. Tell her how it felt to write it.

2. Enjoy an Avalanche of Appreciation about yourself. Look over the following phrases and write at least 25 things you appreciate about yourself.

A. I am... (caring and kind, a nature lover, a good listener, determined, strong, etc.)

B. I can... (write this list, cook, remember birthdays, say thank you, find a bargain, etc.)

C. I know... (I am worth it, I can do this, this program works, etc.)

Share some with your partner. Tell them how that felt.

"Giving thanks, recognizing all the good in your life, is the superpower that moves you into the frequency where beauty and joy and creativity happen."

- Pam Grout,
author of *"Thank and Grow Rich"*

HIGH-WAY 8:
HOPE FOR THE FUTURE

*"Life is not a problem to be solved.
It is a process to be lived."*

- Rick Brown, Th.M.,
CEO at the Institute for Relationship Therapy

One day I fired up my laptop and read the following on my son's Facebook page:

"You'd remember my mom if you ever met her. She has a fiery passion to create better lives for others. She's put herself out there and spent time helping others work through some of the largest social problems in the world: Abuse, Addiction, and the least recognized — lack of Hope."

Some people spend time trying to move out of their own way to make an inch of progress on something they've had on their to-do list for weeks, months, or years. They are afraid that the world will stop them, judge them, or disown them.

My mother doesn't think like that.

When the world comes knocking on my mother's door trying to stop her, she replies, 'I'm sorry, but you must have the wrong person.'

So, I wanted to say thank you to my Mom.

Thank you Mom, for creating Hope, both in myself and in everyone who has been blessed to spend time in your presence."

- Z-man

I still can't read those words without tearing up. Zach captured my life's purpose in a few paragraphs. I have written this and my other books for one reason - **to inspire and ignite hope.**

Do you remember how you felt when you started this book? How strong was your hope muscle then? How strong is it now?

When you started, maybe you felt like I did in 1974 - hungry for answers. Back then I read a book called *Sugar Blues.* **Three times.** I recall one reading where I was feeding myself candy with one hand and holding the book in the other.

The evidence was clear even back then. Sugar was taking me down. But I had no process to get off of it.

What took so long?

Although I wanted to make the break from sugar back then, that first book gave me information but no process and no support. It informed me and alarmed me, but it didn't show me how.

Long ago I realized,

Hope is what happens when you have a process.

You now have a process with 3 Prongs: an easy to follow food program, a comprehensive 8-step empowerment process, and a way to connect with a partner and an ongoing community of support.

It's enough. You're enough.

Your days ahead may be challenging, but you've practiced 8 weeks of new-habits-turned-way-of-life. If you ever lose your way, come back and refresh for another 8 weeks. We'll be here.

In the years since I've been working this process, every day when I awaken it feels like I'm in a different world - a world of greater self-love, joy and peace. I promise you, this world is no illusion. It is real and invites us to a **Get Real** lifestyle. I'm reminded of it every day in emails like this one:

Her Hope in a Poem

As I was finishing this chapter, a 25-year-old Ideal I have grown very close to sent me this:

Hey MK –

Thank you for the wonderful gift of inspiration and accountability that your program offers. It's a lot easier to come out of hiding when you're called to be honest with yourself every day. Here's a poem I wrote as my letter of release. I wanted to share it with you.

> *Hello, My Dear One,*
> *How are you feeling today?*
> *Before you respond,*
> *Send those judgments away.*
>
> *Do you have a head on your shoulders?*
> *And a beating heart?*
> *A thought in your head?*
> *A day to jump start?*

It's easy, you'll see.
There's no other tool you need.
Get up off the ground,
You've already planted the seed.

The shoulds and the coulds
Are a thing of the past
You can and you will
Show up — make it last.

It's time to be honest.
Get real with yourself.
Stand up tall
And take those dreams off the shelf.

Tomorrow is here,
Say goodbye to "Someday."
Stop, take a breath.
Your heart will show you the way.

Close your eyes and see,
You'll feel yourself there.
Don't worry so much
About the when and the where.

What do you feel
Deep in your bones?
Now open the door.
Run towards the unknown.

As you look in the mirror,
Smile and sing.
You're on a journey,
Just open your wings.

- Charlsey H.

I'm so grateful for the hope I hear in Charlsey's words and see in her life. She, and you, are my dreams coming true.

Your next dreams await. You have everything you need. You got this.

Thank you for being coachable. It's been a joy sharing with you.

Blissings,

MK

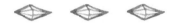

How to Become a Certified 8 to Your IdealWeight Coach

Is your dream to inspire others?

If you feel passionate about the transformational power of this material, I invite you to join us in sharing this message of hope with the world. To find out about becoming a **Certified 8 to Your IdealWeight Coach** and inspiring others from the comfort of your home, contact us at 828-242-9033 or go to coach.8toyouridealweight.com.

Either way, visit us on Facebook or Linkedin or email us at *Ideal@8togreat.com*. We'd love to answer your questions and hear your success stories!

Chapter 5

Additional Resources

IDEALMEALS AND SNACKS

S.A.A.B. Breakfast Bright Ideas

Breakfast is short for "break the fast." It is the meal that gets your metabolism going, and one of the most loving gifts you can give to your body.

I had one Ideal who said she just never had time for breakfast. I asked her if she made breakfast for her children when they were in elementary school.

"Of course!"

"Why?"

"Because I love them."

She made the connection. It is self-loving to take time to eat a relaxing morning meal, even if it means getting up 15 minutes before anyone else in order to do so.

Here are some delicious S.A.A.B. breakfast options:

1. Eggs, hard boiled, scrambled, souffled, etc.

Possible Additions: cheese, mushrooms, onions, tomatoes, green peppers, olives, ham, steak, chicken, turkey, shrimp, crab, salmon, hamburger, sprouts, butter, cream, cottage cheese, goat cheese, feta cheese, bleu cheese, parmesan cheese, ricotta cheese, cheddar cheese, Swiss cheese, spinach, basil, green chilies, dillweed, artichoke hearts, apples, peaches, etc.

2. Cottage Cheese and Fresh Fruit

3. Steel Cut Oats Oatmeal

Possible Additions: apples, bananas, blueberries, raspberries, blackberries, apricots, peaches, pecans, walnuts, almonds, dates, raisins, flax seed, hemp hearts, cinnamon, nutmeg, cloves, ginger, hemp hearts, chia seeds (Note: vanilla extract is not on program)

4. Fruit with Cheese/Nuts

A cheese stick, an apple, and a bag of your favorite tree nuts is great for on the go!

5. Caprese Salad

Fresh mozzarella, tomatoes, basil and olive oil or balsamic vinegar

6. Leftovers from last evening (Who is to say what a "breakfast food" is?)

S.A.A.B. Love-My-Lunch Options

1. Extra Extra: Grill extra chicken or steak at dinner tonight and have the leftovers for lunch tomorrow!

2. Grilled Chicken Salad on romaine lettuce with fruit (strawberries) and pecans and avocado added to taste

3. Cottage Cheese and Fruit with some fresh or leftover veggies

4. Shell-less Tacos in a Bowl with tomatoes, onions, avocado, shredded romaine lettuce, cheese, sour cream, green peppers, grilled chicken or steak, taco sauce packet.

5. Chicken Salad using a rotisserie chicken from the store; add guacamole and/or mayo (low sugar or homemade), halved grapes, walnuts, celery, salt and pepper

6. Caprese Salad: sliced tomato, sliced fresh mozzarella (round), 1 T. Balsamic vinegar.

7. Veggie Tray Treat - buy the tray on Monday and divide it into small sandwich bags for the week. Then portion cheese and/or rotisserie chicken and/or nuts for a perfect "bag" lunch.

8. Go Bowl-ing! Drive through a fast food place and get their grilled chicken or burger in a bowl with NO bread but with all the toppings: lettuce, tomato, onion, cheese, etc. Because they often use processed cheese, have a cheese stick handy to cut up and add. You can also get small packets of guacamole that stay well in a baggie with some ice for a few hours until lunch time. Read the labels!

9. Egg or a Tuna Salad with canned tuna, low sugar or homemade mayo, diced celery, hard-boiled eggs, lemon juice and freshly ground pepper. Serve an apple on the side.

10. Roast Beef Wrap made with sliced roast beef and horseradish or guacamole (lettuce) wrap with tomatoes and cheese.

11. Chicken and Pineapple Wrap - This is a (lettuce) wrap with optional onion and Swiss cheese.

12. Fast Food Option #1: Jimmy John's Unwiches (Lettuce Wraps) - take your pick!

13. Fast Food Option #2: Pei Wei Asian Diner's Vietnamese Chicken Salad Wraps (So good you don't miss the sauce!)

14. Fast Food Option #3: Panda Express Mushroom Chicken or Broccoli Beef or Shanghai Angus Steak. You can get them in little carryout boxes.

15. Fast Food Option #4: Subway Double Chicken Chop Chop Salad. Add avocado, cheese and oil and vinegar dressing for some fun flavor.

16. **Fast Food Option #5: Veggie Delight Sub** - without the bread.

17. **Fast Food Option #6: Pizza from Anywhere** - Just ditch the crust.

18. **Fast Food Option #7: Chipotle Burrito Bowl** - Ask for chicken with fajita veggies, lettuce, tomatoes, guacamole and sour cream.

19. **Fast Food Option #8:** A Burger from anywhere with no bun - have them add cheese, lettuce, tomatoes, onion, mustard, pickle, and you add your own ketchup (2 g of sugar per packet)

20. **Fast Food Option #9:** McDonald's bacon and eggs - served all day.

21. **Spring Mix Salads** - Early in the week get a box of Spring Mix at Sam's Club or Costco. Have any of the following you enjoy on hand: cucumbers, red onion, cherry tomatoes, small peppers, avocados, shredded cheese and shredded almonds. Each day, add a different meat. Needs very little dressing if the ingredients are fresh. Make it in the evening and grab it to go in the morning.

22. **Spinach Salad with Scallops** - If you're lucky like I was, you'll find a restaurant that has these to go with strawberries, guacamole and sliced almonds. A little bit of (not cheap but delicious) heaven!!!

For S.A.A.B. recipe ideas for the evening meal, go to **www.8toyouridealweight.com/recipes4life.**

S.A.A.B. Savory Snacks

Snacks are important in the S.A.A.B. program. Hunger is not our friend. This scientifically supported truth has even sprouted its own word: Hangry!

According to researchers, when we're hungry our blood sugar levels drop. This can make it hard to concentrate, or we may start to drop things or forget what we were doing. A small healthy snack can turn that around.

Meanwhile, treating yourself to a delicious snack can lift your spirits while keeping your metabolism revved, which normalizes blood sugar and helps you release extra weight faster!

Some Great S.A.A.B. Snacks:

- *Harvest Snaps Snapea Crisps*
- *1 Date and 6 Pecans*
- *5-6 Mary's Gone Crackers and 5-6 Almonds*
- *Toasted Almonds (check sugar on side of pkg)*
- *A Cheese Stick*
- *A Handful of Pistachios or Macadamias or Cashews or Pecans*
- *Walnuts and Cheese*
- *Apples, Oranges, Pears, Plums, Mangos, etc.*
- *Apples with Cheese*
- *Tomatoes and Fresh Mozzarella*
- *Celery sticks and Carrots*
- *Veggies and Hummus (watch the portions)*
- *Green and Red Peppers*
- *Mango and Avocado Salsa*

- *Edamame (watch portions)*
- *Grapes or Frozen Grapes*
- *Frozen Bananas with Nuts*
- *Frozen Pineapple*
- *Avocado and Cottage Cheese with Smoked Salmon or pre-cooked Shrimp*
- *Celery and Peanut-free Nut Butters like Nuttzo*
- *Shaved Roast Beef around a Cheese Stick or slice of Cheese*
- *Watermelon, Cantaloupe, Honeydew, Mango*
- *Hard-boiled Eggs*
- *Kale Chips*
- *Meat Sticks (check sugar content)*
- *Pumpkin seeds*
- *Radishes with Salt*
- *Sunflower Seeds*
- *Baked Sweet Potato Chips (shave and bake your own!)*
- *Plain Yogurt, add your own fresh fruit*
- *Cottage Cheese with a fresh Peach, Pear, or Pineapple and Nuts*
- *Deviled Eggs*
- *Kind Bars with 6 g of sugar or less - Nuts and Spices, Dark Chocolate Almond Mint and Dark Chocolate Mocha Almond*

The S.A.A.B. Foods FAQ's

When asked, "May I have the following foods?" The answer is, you are in charge of your life and this program. For those on this program, here are the foods we recommend avoiding and some questionable ones that are on program.

Again, thank you for trusting us to be your guides, not just in food but in freedom, fulfillment, and feeling good. The S.A.A.B. plan and The 8 High-Ways will get us where we want to go, feeling passionate and powerful again!

Gratefully,

MK

FOODS FAQ's: Are these foods on my 8-week program?

- Almond Flour? *No*
- Arrowroot Powder? *Yes*
- Bacon? *Yes - see label and count sugars*
- Buckwheat? *No*
- Cocoa? *Yes, if it's 100 percent cocoa.*
- Canola Oil or Coconut oil or Sunflower Oil? *Yes - watch portions*
- Carob? *Yes*
- Chia seeds? *Yes*
- Coconut Flour? *No*

- Coffees and Teas? *Yes - any sugar added must be added by you*
- Cream Cheese? *Yes - see label and count sugars*
- Dates? *Yes*
- Dijon Mustard? *Yes*
- Flax seeds? *Yes*
- Fruit juice? *No*
- Gluten Free Breads/Cereal/Pasta? *No*
- Sugar free gum? *Yes - watch portions*
- Hummus? *Yes - watch portions*
- Mary's Gone Crackers? *Yes - (made of seeds and nuts)*
- Mayonnaise? *Yes, see label and count sugars or make your own. Here's a great recipe:*

  http://tinyurl.com/hg4f7r5

  > *1 egg, 2 T lemon juice,*
  > *1/4 c. light (NOT virgin) olive oil,*
  > *1/2 tsp. dry mustard,*
  > *1/2 tsp. salt*

- Paleo Bread? *No*
- Paleo Ice Cream? *No*
- Popcorn? *No*
- Quinoa? *Yes*
- Salt? *Yes - watch portions*
- Snow Peas? *Yes - watch portions*
- Sour Cream? *Yes*
- Stevia? *No*
- Tahini? *Yes*
- Vanilla Extract? *No (alcohol). Try Vanilla Bean Powder.*
- Yogurt? *Yes, if plain. Add your own fruit.*

How to Stay on Program While You Travel/Vacation

Q: Can I go "off program" while I'm on vacation?

A: Yes. You're in charge of how quickly you release your weight. Be clear with yourself that no guilt is allowed, and that you will not compare your results to those who stayed on program over that time period.

Or you can learn how to happily stay on program (which is amazingly easy) while on vacation using the tips below. Remember, this is not a diet. It's a fun and filling way to Eat-For-Life.

Here are some tips that have helped me stay true to my goals while thoroughly enjoying my work trips and vacations:

1. Pack Snacks. I pack two small packets of my fave crackers and almonds for every day I'll be on the road. Instead of packing one big package, use small plastic baggies and allow yourself to eat one every 5-6 hours between meals.

2. Eat breakfast. Every hotel has breakfast now. Choose eggs or oatmeal and meat and fruit. You will be full within 10 minutes - I guarantee it.

3. Have an "emergency" fast food decision already made. What can you eat at fast food places that will not be full of sugar?

4. Drink lots of water. Flying is especially dehydrating. Thirst can feel like hunger.

5. Get extra sleep. This is always important, especially if changing time zones.

6. Get really good at asking for what you want, from "dressing on the side" to "no need to bring us bread," to "please remove the snacks from my hotel room immediately."

7. Refrain from alcohol. It's just 8 weeks. Perrier or tonic water can look (and feel) very sophisticated!

8. Walk the stairs in a hotel if no workout rooms are available. There's your fitness for the day!

9. Make extra efforts to "Self-Comfort" such as: Get a massage, get a manicure/pedi, take your softest throw blanket, order room service, make quiet time for reading, music or a bubble bath, travel by uber or a limo, and do your best not to touch your luggage!

I travel for my work and play. Getting comfortable with eating on the road has been vital to my making permanent changes in my "Loving-My-Lifestyle."

How to Stay on the S.A.A.B. Program When Eating Out

1. Be selective - choose your restaurant wisely. *(When I'm invited to go to a new restaurant, I google their menu and make sure they have foods I want.)*

2. Ask questions and be very clear on how you want your food prepared. *(See Meg Ryan's famous pie scene in "Harry Met Sally".)*

3. Inform the server you do not want any bread or chips on the table as soon as you get there.

4. Ask for water right away.

5. Ask for all sauces and dressings on the side.

6. Ask for extra avocado or tomato on the side.

7. Always take your crackers/almonds/fave snack with you.

8. Consider having unsweetened tea, hot water, a cup of coffee or a piece of sugar free gum if your companions are having dessert (although fewer and fewer of them do!)

9. Ask for any sandwich or taco to be served in a bowl with no bun or tortilla. Even McDonald's won't be surprised by the request.

10. If you're at an event and pizza is the only offering, just eat the toppings. And really "chew on" all the compliments you'll be getting from the participants on how *great* you look!

How to Break Through a Plateau

When faced with a scale number that doesn't reward you, even though you stayed on program, take a deep breath...

When I was 40 I had my "miracle baby." I had gained 42 pounds. After his birth, I lost 6 pounds. I hung onto those other 36 pounds *for six weeks.* Then one day, it happened. I released 14 pounds in two days, and the rest over the next month.

Why did my body hang onto that weight? It had nothing to do with what I was eating. Guilt would have been such a burden to add to all the new stressors of being Mom to a newborn! As we look at "scale surprises," it's good to remember to check for any internal resistance to release.

How Carrie Broke Through

When Carrie joined the program she was at the top of her game. . . at work. Her weight had been steadily increasing with the stress of her new promotion. Handling that as well as her daughter's soccer practices was a challenge. She was grateful when her husband said he'd take some extra carpooling duties so she could take the **8 to Your IdealWeight** course.

Carrie was thrilled when she released her first 10 and then 20 pounds. She acknowledged that she had no idea it could be this easy or fun to eat well. But then she noticed her scale numbers hitting a plateau. After four weeks of eating on program with no release, she contacted me for a coaching session.

I listened and affirmed she was following the program, and then asked her to write 10 completions for this sentence:

The worst thing about reaching my IdealWeight would be...

After only three sentences, she had solved the mystery.

"It hit me between the eyes when I wrote, 'The worst thing about reaching my IdealWeight would be making my sister feel bad.' No wonder I was dreading the family reunion."

I asked her to explain.

"My younger sister's had a tough time of it. Her marriage ended last year and now it looks like she's going to be downsized. We've always both been heavy and I was feeling guilty that I not only had a great husband, job and kids, but now I was also going to look great. . . Well, I didn't want to make her feel worse."

We reviewed the **8 to your IdealWeight** teaching on guilt:

Guilt about stepping outside your moral values is healthy.

Guilt about anything else is not.

I invited her to entertain the possibility that her new slimmer and trimmer torso might inspire and ignite her sister with the much needed angergy to get off high-sugar foods herself. We agreed that whether it did or did not, she could release trying to rescue her sister from the pain of reality.

The next week she released four pounds and she had a great time at the reunion.

5 Break-Through-Your-Barriers Questions

If you're in the midst of a plateau, look over the following 5 questions to see which one speaks to you. Eventually, you can do each of them; but start with the one you feel strongest about, whether it is the strongest resistance or the strongest attraction.

A. What or who is weighing me down these days?

B. Who would be the most upset or jealous if I reached my IdealWeight?

C. What weakness of mine sometimes makes me feel "not enough"?

D. What is my self-talk saying to me on my hardest days?

E. What would I need to do/be to deserve happiness?

After you journal an answer to one or more of these questions, there's no need to take immediate action unless you feel led to do so. The awareness itself will bring what was hiding in the dark corners of your mind into the light. When we are willing to see what we have been hiding from ourselves, what we see will motivate and empower us.

Meanwhile, here are some more pointers on how plateaus work...

1. Plateaus happen to everyone and they can last 3-4 weeks. The most important thing to do is stay the course and avoid giving your power away to the scale numbers. Check in regularly with your partner and coach to be reminded of your personal goals and dreams!

2. Record what you eat and drink for 24 hours and share your food log with your Coach. Be sure you haven't slipped back into old habits. Pay attention to details.

3. If you're clear that you've been 100% on the S.A.A.B. program, and after 2 weeks are still not releasing, **try the following for three days in a row** and weigh yourself every 3 days:

> A. Vary your food choices. Add half an avocado each day, cut down to 1/2 a Kind bar each day, or simply eat lunch for breakfast and breakfast for lunch.

The website **www.emeals.com** is a great place to find low-sugar recipes.

> B. Drink 6-8 oz. of water before each meal. Whether it's 30 seconds or 30 minutes before does not matter.

4. If you're not seeing a difference after a week of these changes, vary your movement. Changing the type or amount of movement/exercise you do can "wake up" a sleepy metabolism.

5. Keep track of your bowel movements. Daily is best, but you need to be releasing at least every other day. If not, add fiber (i.e. flaxseed), drink more water, take a detox bath, and/or talk with your coach or partner.

6. If after 4 weeks of experimenting with these various techniques, your weight is still not decreasing, check with your medical professional. It could be a thyroid or other medical issue that can be diagnosed and easily remedied.

Movies that Move Us

What are some movies that have "moved" you?

To get myself feeling and healing, I love to see true story films, for real life is so amazing and exciting that it doesn't need embellishing. Some of my favorite true stories are:

- *Big Miracle*
- *(The) Blind Side*
- *Eat Pray Love*
- *Erin Brockovich*
- *Freedom Writers*
- *Helen Keller*
- *(The) Help***
- *Hoosiers*
- *McFarland USA*
- *Million Dollar Arm*
- *Miracles from Heaven*
- *Invincible*
- *October Sky*
- *Pursuit of Happyness*
- *Remember the Titans*
- *Rudy*
- *Stand and Deliver*
- *Suffragette*
- *We Bought a Zoo*

**(While not a true story of one woman, The Help was, I believe, true for a generation, and is incredibly powerful.)*

Some of my favorite fiction films for helping me feel my feelings are:

- *Chocolat*
- *Dragonfly*
- *Field of Dreams*
- *Salmon Fishing in Yemen*
- *Whose Life Is It Anyway*

For more films and book suggestions, go to www.idealweight.com/recipes4life.

ACKNOWLEDGMENTS

To my Excellent Editing Team8s - Barb Fritzler, Julie Delkamiller, Amy Krance-Wendt, Mary Beth Helgens, Dana Lyn, Betsy Blondin and Christina Auch - Thank you so much for helping me put this movement into a manual.

To my John-of-the-Heart: Sweetheart, thank you for blessing my life with so much love and laughter, as well as nourishing me with the kind of support I have always dared to dream of. You are my teacher, my best friend and my forty-ever love. XO

To Jim Schneider: Thank you O Courageous One, for the email full of gratitude that was the snowflake that started this avalanche of love. So grateful to have you as a Coach and a friend.

To the rest of my Charter Group of Coaches, great gratitude for trusting me then and continuing to share the message today: Sue Fitzgerald, Patty Stuever, Peggy Hinman, Beth Schmitt, Mary Beth Helgens, and Bonita Yoder.

To Dr. Michelle Robin: How can I ever thank you for that gentle push to go to the next level of health and wellness? You are changing the world one person at a time with your love and light, and we all join in a chorus of gratitude!

To my Dear and Daring Dana Lyn: Thank you for your truth - in editing my writings and calming my fears. Your gentle guidance and strong-as-steel friendship keep me going and growing.

AUTHOR BIO

A former binge eater and domestic violence survivor, at the age of 34 MK Mueller put together a program for her own recovery and began a support group in her home called *"Taking Care of Me."* Almost overnight the group outgrew her living room and she became an international speaker and trainer, working with individuals, schools, health care organizations, and Fortune 500 companies.

Today her first book, **Taking Care of Me: The Habits of Happiness**, and her award-winning *8 to Great: The Powerful Process for Positive Change*, are being taught by thousands of Certified Trainers around the world. Together, they built the foundation for the acclaimed *8 to Great* curriculum for schools and businesses as well as the life-changing *8 to Your IdealWeight* program.

These days MK is loving life in Southwest Florida as a **TEDx** presenter, a writer, a keynote speaker, a pickleball player, the mother of two amazing young adults - Joanna and Zach - and the devoted partner of John of the Heart.

Other Books by MK Mueller available at www.8togreat.com:

8 to Great: The Powerful Process for Positive Change
Taking Care of Me: The Habits of Happiness
Becoming a Magnificent Manifaster